HEALTH IN OUR TIME?

UNIVERSITY OF LIVERPOOL
FACULTY OF MEDICINE

THE INAUGURAL
DUNCAN MEMORIAL LECTURE

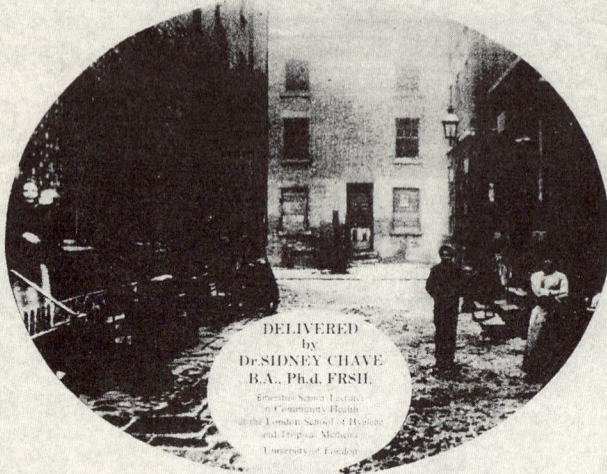

DELIVERED
by
Dr. SIDNEY CHAVE
B.A., Ph.d, FRSH,

Emeritus Senior Lecturer
in Community Health
at the London School of Hygiene
and Tropical Medicine
University of London

DUNCAN OF LIVERPOOL
SOME LESSONS FOR TODAY

at 5.00 p.m. on Wednesday, 23rd November, 1983

in the Henry Cohen Lecture Theatre, Duncan Building, Royal Liverpool Hospital
(entry off Daulby Street)

Supported by the Health Education Council
Open to the Public

DESIGNED BY PAUL SMITH, SECOND YEAR GRAPHICS, MABEL FLETCHER COLLEGE.

Health in Our Time?

The William Henry Duncan Memorial Lectures

Carnegie Publishing, 1997

Published by Carnegie Publishing Ltd
18 Maynard Street, Preston PR2 2AL

© respective contributors and journals, 1997

Printed by Bookcraft (Bath) Ltd

British Library Cataloguing-in-Publication Data
A catalogue record for this book is available from
the British Library

ISBN 1-85936-056-4

Contents

Acknowledgements

The Duncan lectures have been tremendously successful due not only to the choice of speakers and their topics, but also due to the efforts of a number of people within the University of Liverpool. Heather Ainscough in the Dean's office of the Faculty of Medicine has provided excellent administrative support, and ensured that the post-lecture celebrations have been very enjoyable.

Dr Gillian Maudsley and Dr Mary Jane Platt have both been enthusiastic publicists and through their efforts the Duncan lectures have been well advertised both within and without the University. Thanks also to Paul Blackburn, Alistair Livingstone and Chris West for tape recording the lectures, and to the Public Health Department secretaries for transcribing the tapes to help the speakers produce their papers for publication.

Introduction

Welcome to the first volume of the Duncan lectures. This is a record of a lecture series which began in 1983 and ranges far and wide through territory which makes up the New Public Health. (Ashton and Seymour 1988, Ashton 1995). The material is both a historical record and a contemporary reference to a discipline which has recently re-emerged from a dark age of bio-medical reductionism which threatened to eclipse over 100 years of experience in the practice of 'the science and art of preventing disease. prolonging life and promoting physical health and efficiency through organised community efforts for the sanitation of the environment, the education of the individual in the principles of personal hygiene, the organisation of medical and nursing service for the early diagnosis and preventive treatment of disease, and the development of the social machinery which will ensure to every individual in the community a standard of living adequate for the maintenance of health' (Winslow 1920).

The idea of an annual public health lecture in recognition of the country's first Medical Officer of Health, open to the public, owes much to the influence of the late Dr Sidney Chave of the London School of Hygiene and Tropical Medicine. For many of us studying at the School in the 1970s Sidney was an inspirational force in drawing on historical perspectives to understand current public health challenges and in connecting to the public in imaginative ways to further the cause of public health. This was very much in the tradition of Duncan himself whose survey of the sanitary conditions in Liverpool led to his publishing a pamphlet on the subject, to public lectures at the Liverpool Royal Institution, to his leading role in the establishment of the Liverpool Health of Towns Association in 1845 and his notorious stream of agitating and campaigning letters to London in the cause of sanitary reform. In addition to Sidney Chave's prolific publications, the John Snow pub in Soho and the Jeremy Bentham in Bloomsbury are two enduring souvenirs of his imagination and populist instincts (Warren and Francis 1987). It was therefore fitting that Sidney Chave delivered the first Duncan lecture on the topic of 'Duncan of Liverpool - some lessons for today' to a packed Cohen auditorium in the Liverpool Medical School. In this Sidney set another precedent, for in the ensuing years the lecture has established itself as one of the most popular eponymous university lectures, regularly attracting 200-300 people from a wide range of professional and lay backgrounds on cold December evenings.

From the outset the intention was for the lectures to visit the major domains that impact on public health as so clearly evidenced in McKeown's seminal Rock Carling lecture in 1976 on the role of medicine - genetics, lifestyles, food, occupation and the environment and medical and social care supported by appropriate education, training and research (McKeown 1976). The result has been a rich menu of offerings from some of the major contemporary thinkers and practitioners in the field of public health. It seemed timely to publish the first volume of lectures to coincide with the 150th anniversary of Duncan's appointment as Medical Officer of Health in Liverpool. These offerings remind us too of the essentially practical and political nature of public health and of Virchow's well-known aphorism that 'medicine is social science and politics is nothing else but medicine on a large scale' (Virchow 1848). When that message has been lost or forgotten medicine has found itself in some dire cul-de-sacs where it has more in common with accountancy than with the great humanitarian and shared task which it can be at its best.

Finally I would like to acknowledge the contribution of Dr David Player who as Director of the Health Education Council before its demise in 1986 lent his support to the lecture series, and to Dr Spencer Hagard who continued to support it from the successor Health Education Authority. Throughout this first era of lectures they have also enjoyed the active support of the Mersey Regional Health Authority, later the North West Regional Health Authority and the National Health Service North West, the Liverpool District Health Authority, the University of Liverpool Department of Public Health and successive Deans of Medicine at Liverpool

John Ashton
Liverpool
January 1997

References

1. Ashton, J. and Seymour, H. (1988) The New Public Health (Open University Press, 1988)
2. Ashton, J. 'Recalling the Medical Officer of Health' Health Promotion 1989 Vol.3 No.4 pp.413-419.
3. Ashton, J. A vision of health for the North West (Liverpool Public Health Observatory, 1995)
4. McKeown, T. The Role of Medicine: Dream, Mirage or Nemesis? (The Nuffield Provincial Hospitals Trust, 1976)
5. Virchow, R.L.K. Die Medizinische Reform (1848) p.2. Quoted in Sigerist, H.E. Medicine and Human Welfare (New Haven, Yale University Press, 1941) p.93.
6. Warren, M. and Francis, H. Recalling the Medical Officer of Health (King Edward's Hospital Fund for London, 1987)
7. Winslow, C.E.A. 'The Untilled Fields of Public Health', Science 1920 51:23

Duncan of Liverpool –
and some lessons for today*

S. P. W. Chave, London School of Hygiene and Tropical Medicine,
Community Medicine, Vol. 6, No. 1 (February 1984)

I want to begin this lecture not with Duncan, but with the man who more than anyone else was responsible for starting it all; the man who those of us who work in the broad fields of public and community health still look on as our godfather – I refer, of course, to Edwin Chadwick. Chadwick's long life spanned 90 years of the last century. He lived through the battles of Waterloo and Peterloo; the Corn Laws and the Crimean War; he saw the Great Exhibition and the coming of the Great Western Railway. All these events, and what they represented, must form the unspoken, but assumed background against which we should see the life and work of William Henry Duncan.

But to continue with Chadwick, in his well-known *Report on the Sanitary Condition of the Labouring Population* he wrote the following paragraph:

> That for the general means necessary to prevent disease, it would be good economy to appoint a district medical officer, independent of private practice, with the securities of special qualifications, and responsibilities to initiate sanitary measures and reclaim the execution of the law.

This was the moment of conception of the Medical Officer of Health – the MOH. And that was in 1842. Five years later, after a somewhat troubled gestation, he came to birth in Liverpool in the person of William Henry Duncan. But why Liverpool? and why Duncan? Why indeed!

Liverpool is well-known as a famous port with a long history. It thrived on the slave trade, being one of the ports of call on the triangular route on which that revolting commerce was based. Then later as industrial development took place in Lancashire in the nineteenth century, Liverpool became the principal port both for the import of raw materials and for the export of manufactured goods across the world. But Liverpool manufactured very little for itself, rather it was a staging post in this two-way traffic.

So what characterized the working population in the town at that time, and what distinguished it from the main Lancashire towns, was that it was composed not of workers employed in factories and mills getting regular wages, small as they might be, but that it consisted very largely of unskilled casual labourers

---

* The inaugural Duncan Memorial Lecture delivered in the University of Liverpool on 23 December 1983.

without regular employment. It was casual labourers who came to Liverpool to build the docks, and it was casual labourers, the dockers, who loaded and unloaded the ships. Theirs was a particularly vulnerable occupation, for when the ships came in there was work for them to do, but when there were no ships, they stood idle, and any down-turn in trade brought unemployment and destitution. All this meant that they had very little money with which to obtain the essentials of life in terms of food, clothing and shelter. In particular, they could afford only the meanest housing accommodation and that is exactly what they got.

Houses were hastily built without regard to suitability of soil or site, for water supply or sanitation. Hundreds of dwellings were packed together in narrow courts with an opening at one end only. And the people were packed together inside them, literally from cellar to attic. Accumulations of refuse and soil-heaps, and evil-smelling and over-flowing cess-pools were common features of this unwholesome environment.

Dirt, disease and malnourishment flourished. Chief among the diseases were typhoid and typhus, which had not by then been distinguished and were known together as 'the fever'. There was dysentery, scarlet fever, measles and, of course, tuberculosis – 'the captain of the men of death'. Then there was cholera which was the Victorian equivalent of the medieval Black Death and which, since the successful introduction of vaccination, had replaced smallpox as the epidemic disease most to be feared.

Such then was Liverpool in the year 1840. The picture can be summed up not in a word, but in a figure; that figure was 36. The annual death rate in Liverpool was 36 per 1000 and that was the highest in the country. Liverpool was, in fact, the most unhealthy town in the kingdom, hence Liverpool. But why Duncan?

Historians are in some ways like epidemiologists. As epidemiologists, when investigating the occurrence of disease, we are trained to look for three factors, time, place and person, as pointers to the origin of the outbreak. So does the historian; when seeking to understand the occurrence of some historical event, he looks for the relevant circumstances at the time and in the place where the event occurred, but then there is generally the person who in some way, perhaps through speech, thought or action, or perhaps all three, was instrumental in bringing the event to pass.

So it was in Liverpool at the time, and in the circumstances that we have been considering. Which brings us to William Henry Duncan.

Frazer tells us that Duncan was a Liverpolitan born and bred. He was born in Seel Street, then one of the more salubrious areas of the town, in 1805, the year of the Battle of Trafalgar – an event itself significant to Liverpool for it re-opened the sea-lanes to maritime trade once again. Young William was the third son and the fifth child of his father, a merchant whose business was in the town. His mother, who came from a clerical family, was a Scot from Dumfries.

We believe he attended school in the town after which he went up to

Edinburgh to study medicine. He graduated MD at the age of 25 with a thesis written in impeccable Latin entitled *De Ventris In Reliquum Corpus Potestate*. While in Edinburgh he would certainly have heard about the work and writings of Johann Peter Frank and his system of 'Medicinischen Polizey', or medical police. In this massive work Frank argued with great cogency, and showed in great detail, how the state could, and indeed should, assume responsibility for the health and welfare of all its citizens, and should ensure this by regulating their every behaviour from the cradle to the grave. Frank's work was held in high esteem by the Scottish academics.

But the idea of medical police was not to the taste of the English with their 'Victorian values' where 'laisser-faire', sturdy independence, and unfettered private enterprise was the accepted dogma.

Only gradually under the unanswerable case for state intervention to control private interests in favour of the public weal, which was advanced first, and unsuccessfully, by Chadwick, and somewhat later, but more diplomatically by Simon, did this characteristically English philosophy begin to break down. But all that lay in the future.

The seed of this idea has been sown in Duncan's mind and he returned to his native soil to tend its development.

On his return to Liverpool, he immediately began to take an active part in the professional and social life of the town. He took up residence at 54 Rodney Street, which became the family home, and commenced to practice. He joined the Liverpool Medical Institution (the subscription list shows that he subscribed the sum of five pounds towards the erection of the present building in Hope Street). In 1837 he became President of the Liverpool Medical Society. Shortly after he was appointed Lecturer in Medical Jurisprudence in the Medical School at the Royal Institution. In addition to all this he became a member of the Athenaeum and was also a regular attender at the meetings of the Liverpool Literary and Philosophical Society; and this was to prove to be important later on.

But let us now turn to his professional life. As I said, he took up private practice at first among the Liverpolitans of his own class. In this he soon became a successful young practitioner with a circle of patients among the well-to-do – and there was nothing remarkable about that. But then, for his own reasons, he took a post as an honorary physician to the Dispensaries which catered for the sick poor, working first at the North Dispensary and then later at the South Dispensary which was located at 1 Upper Parliament Street. These Dispensaries were supported in part by the parish and in part by charity.

It was here that Duncan first came face to face with the twin-related evils that had already confronted Chadwick, namely, dire sickness and abject poverty. There is no doubt that Duncan was moved by what he saw at first hand in those overcrowded hovels and insanitary courts. This was the first step along the path which was to take him into public health.

When in 1832 cholera struck Liverpool for the first time, he was working among both sections of the community – the upper class Liverpolitans and the working class Liverpudlians. He was immediately struck by how much greater were the casualties of the epidemic among the poor and overcrowded, than they were among the better off and better housed. So he wrote a paper on this for the Liverpool Medical Gazette, the first of a number of such papers that he contributed to his local journal. In these papers he invariably referred to the insanitary conditions prevailing in the poorer parts of the town.

When in 1840, the House of Commons Select Committee on the Health of Towns visited Liverpool, Duncan appeared before them as a witness and gave evidence on what he called 'the bad pre-eminence of the worst population density in the land'. He reported that one third of the working class lived in Liverpool's typical narrow and airless courts and one eighth lived in underground cellars. The public lodging houses, of which there were hundreds, were packed to the doors often with thirty people sleeping in a cellar. Only four of the twenty miles of streets in the working class areas were sewered. No wonder, he said, the fevers were 'rampant'.

The Committee were obviously impressed. They recorded his evidence in their proceedings, but no action followed. Later in the same year he submitted a written report in the same terms in answer to an enquiry by the Poor Law Commission, which had been initiated by Chadwick. Here he cited the example of one court of twelve houses where, because of the complete absence of any kind of drainage, the whole court was permanently inundated with filth, and in those twelve houses, he said, there had been no fewer than 63 cases of fever.

This was probably Duncan's first contact with Chadwick who was then Secretary, and Chief Executive Officer, to the Poor Law Commission. There were to be many more such contacts in the years to follow.

It is worth making the point here that Duncan shared the work at the Dispensaries with several other colleagues, all of whom must have seen the same destitution, degradation and distress in the districts which were served by the Dispensaries, but only one of them did anything about it, and that was William Henry Duncan.

By now Duncan had twice reported to official enquiries about the mean and stinking conditions in which so many of his fellow townsfolk were compelled to live, and die. It seems that he was not satisfied simply to continue to be a witness to others, he now began to be active in this cause in his own right.

He had by this time marshalled a body of evidence concerning the unhealthiness of Liverpool; he now re-organized and expanded this material and used it to prepare two lectures under the title of 'The Physical Causes of the High Rate of Mortality in Liverpool'. And he delivered these two lectures not, as you might expect, to the Medical Society, not to the doctors, but to the Literary and Philosophical Society, of which, as I mentioned earlier, he was a member.

Why did he choose this audience of lay people in preference to his medical colleagues? Almost certainly, to bring what he had to say to a wider audience, and to an audience which included some of the best educated and most influential people in the town. Good tactics this – and one which we might do well to follow when we have a case to make.

The lectures achieved what he had hoped; they were widely reported round the town and aroused considerable local interest. Duncan then followed this up by publishing the text of the lectures in pamphlet form, under the same title.

The pamphlet, better described as a booklet, consisted of 76 printed pages. In it he set out fully the mortality in Liverpool and made some comparisons with other areas. Some of these comparisons might well make our modern statisticians' hair stand on end, because he was not always comparing like with like and knew nothing about standardization. But then, he had not the benefits, and delights, of Bradford Hill's little book on *Medical Statistics* to put him on the right lines! So, delving into William Farr's handiwork at the General Register Office he showed that the average age of death in the County of Wiltshire was 36.5 years whereas in Liverpool it was only 19 years. He then went on to explain this high mortality in terms of the prevailing theory of the miasma. This held that the fevers were caused by foul air rising from the decomposition, the putrefaction, of organic matter and waste. This view was held by the great majority of his colleagues in the medical profession; it was the view held by the sanitary reformers; it was the view held by Chadwick himself. Indeed, Chadwick's own work was taken to give proof to the theory, for it was in the most overcrowded, unsewered and unventilated quarters that the incidence of the fevers invariably reached its peak. This was the basic premise on which Chadwick had built his 'Sanitary Idea' which was to infuse the Public Health movement for the next fifty years, and which led to his simple and sovereign remedy for the prevention of fevers, namely, a drainage system backed by a supply of running water to flush away the filth and disease-causing odours deriving from it.

Duncan, in pursuing his own inquiries in Liverpool, reached the same general conclusion as to the cause, but he gave greater weight to what he called 'vitiated air' derived from respiring human beings. This, he claimed, became particularly dangerous when associated with the effluvia arising from putrefaction, and more especially so when confined in enclosed spaces. However, as for Chadwick, so for Duncan, the remedy was the same – reduction in overcrowding, improved ventilation and an effective system of drainage.

The publication of the pamphlet aroused much discussion in the town, as well as some mixed feelings. There were those, whom we might call the local patriots, who accused him of denigrating 'the good old town' as they called it. A local surgeon was bold enough to try to refute Duncan's statistics – but he had not read Bradford Hill either! Duncan went back to the Registrar General's Reports yet again and from these he showed that the annual death rate in Liverpool was 1 in 28 persons, whereas in Birmingham it was 1 in 36 and in London it was 1 in 37.

By all the yardsticks Liverpool really was the most unhealthy town in the country and, by now, largely due to Duncan, the town knew it. Things began to move.

In 1845, as a result of growing feeling, the Mayor called a public meeting which was addressed at some length by Duncan, the object of which was to form a Health of Towns Association, similar to the one which had been set up in London in the previous year. Its object was:

> to bring the subject of sanitary reform under the notice of every class of the community, to diffuse sound principles as widely as possible by meetings, lectures, and publications, and especially to give information on all points connected with the sanitary condition of Liverpool, and the means of improving it.

The Association was formed and soon won the support of many of the prominent people in the town.

This led directly to the next step which came in the following year when the Council promoted a private Bill in Parliament seeking wide powers to pursue a programme of sanitary reform and, most significantly, the Bill included a clause empowering the Council to appoint a Medical Officer of Health.

The Bill passed through Parliament without demur as the Liverpool Sanitary Act 1846. It was a milestone in the history of English public health, for it was the first comprehensive sanitary Act to be passed into law, and it gave authority for the appointment of an MOH. It is worth the comment, that when a year later the City of London copied the example of Liverpool and obtained similar powers also to appoint an MOH, it advertised the post, received 20 applications and appointed the youngest of them, namely, John Simon.

But in the case of Liverpool there was only one possible candidate. The Council went through the motions of setting up a special committee to consider the appointment of an MOH. The Committee immediately offered Duncan the post and he immediately accepted. On 1 January 1847 the Secretary of State confirmed the appointment, as the Act required, and on that day William Henry Duncan became the first Medical Officer of Health in British history. Liverpool deserves the credit for having made this appointment but then Liverpool, above all other towns in the country, needed him the most.

Duncan was aged 42; on his appointment his salary was £300 a year with the right to continue with his private practice. However, he soon found this arrangement incompatible with his official duties. For one thing, he could have found himself in an invidious position if he had had to take action against a landlord who was one of his patients. Moreover, this arrangement did not accord with Chadwick's wishes who had always argued against part-time appointments. So, after a year, the appointment was made full-time at a salary of £750. This despite the opposition of one councillor who thought that the money would be better spent on lime-washing the town, and another who argued strongly that you did not need a doctor to do this job anyway. And how many times since then have we heard that argument!

It is not easy for us to enter into Duncan's feelings on that morning when he went into his office for the first time, because he never told us. He was a somewhat reserved man who wrote little outside his official correspondence and his formal reports. Certainly we know that at the start he had no assistance or support of any kind. It is true that there was Mr Fresh, the Inspector of Nuisances, who was also appointed under the Act, but although he was to work closely with Duncan, he was an independent officer of the Council.

Duncan had no precedents to guide him, no colleagues anywhere in the country with whom he might discuss his problems, his programme or his plans.

Yet he was not altogether without some guide-lines and these were provided, surprisingly enough, by the clause in the Act under which he was appointed. And although the clause is a long one, I want to quote part of it because it was to be an important statement in its own right. It reads:

> It shall be lawful for the said Council to appoint, subject to the approval of one of Her Majesty's Secretaries of State, a legally qualified medical practitioner of skill and experience to inspect and report periodically on the sanitary state of the said borough, to ascertain the existence of diseases, more especially of epidemics increasing the rate of mortality, and to point out the existence of any nuisances or other local causes which are likely to originate and maintain such diseases, and injuriously affect inhabitants of the said borough, and to take cognizance of the fact of the existence of any contagious disease, and so to point out the most efficacious means or checking and preventing the spread of such diseases, and also to point out the most efficient means for the ventilation of churches, chapels, schools, registered lodging houses and other public edifices within the said borough ... and such person shall be called the Medical Officer of Health for the Borough of Liverpool, and it shall be lawful for the said Council to pay such Officer such salary as shall be approved by one of Her Majesty's Principal Secretaries of State.

This, then, was the original job specification of the MOH and, incidentally, it is the first mention of the title of Medical Officer of Health in any Act of Parliament, or indeed, in any official document.

So he had to 'inspect and report' on all matters which might injuriously affect the public health, to advise on such actions which should be taken to deal with them, and to have special regard to infectious diseases. The emphasis laid on the need for proper ventilation of public buildings shows the general acceptance of the theory of the miasma. This clause was to be quoted many times in the years to come.

So perhaps, in our imagination, we can picture Duncan like Saint George as he sallied forth armed with the weapons forged by Chadwick to combat the Monster Miasma. Well a Monster it proved to be, or rather a Hydra, because the Monster was soon shown to be many-headed. For Duncan's luck was out, because the next three years turned out to be the most calamitous in Liverpool's history. It all began with the Irish potato famine. This had started in 1845 with the failure of the potato crop and in the next two years it reached disastrous proportions. Starvation was widespread. Driven by hunger, thousands of Irish peasants migrated to England, and they travelled by way of Liverpool. At times they were being landed at the rate of 900 a day, the fare for standing room on the deck being only sixpence a head.

Duncan reported later to the Council 'that not less than 300,000 Irish have landed in Liverpool. Of these it is estimated that from 60,000 to 80,000 have located themselves amongst us, occupying every nook and cranny of the already overcrowded lodging-houses and forcing their way into cellars of which there are several thousand still remaining in the town.'

The inevitable result of this influx of desperately poor, unwashed and starving people was a massive outbreak of typhus. Within a short time hospitals were packed to the doors with patients lying three to a bed. Emergency accommodation was opened wherever possible. Duncan obtained permission to make use of ships anchored in the docks. And still the cases admitted were exceeded twice over by those for whom no accommodation could be provided. Beyond this there was little that Duncan could do save practise his sanitary principles – remove such cases as he could and cleanse and limewash infected premises and districts.

At the end of the year he estimated that nearly 60,000 people had suffered from fever while a further 40,000 had contracted either diarrhoea or dysentery. There were, he said, 8500 deaths from these causes; smallpox had also occurred and carried off 380 children, while measles had added a similar number to the total. Altogether the toll of deaths from all causes that year amounted to no less than one in 14 of the population of the town. It was the most fatal year in the annals of Liverpool, and it was the first year that Liverpool had had a Medical Officer of Health.

The epidemic subsided in the following year although the death rate from infectious diseases still remained high – a severe outbreak of scarlet fever carried off over 1,500 victims, while tuberculosis accounted for 1,400 more, although there was nothing exceptional about that.

But Duncan's troubles were not over, because in 1849 a family of emigrants arrived by steamer from Dumfries where cholera was raging. Three of these newcomers developed cholera and died within a few days. Then a woman in the same house went down with the disease, and then another, and another and within a short time the outbreak was spreading in all directions. It cut through the crowded populations in those courts and tenements like the sickle of death. Duncan again instituted his sanitary programme, and, in addition, he introduced a system of medical visitors who went round the affected areas seeking out cases in their early stages and starting such treatment as was then available. But at times the outbreak reached overwhelming proportions. At its peak there were over 500 deaths in a week and mass burials in open pits were resorted to, as in the days of the plague. Altogether there were over 5000 deaths from cholera that year.

After those three crisis years in which the new Medical Officer of Health must have felt himself to have been well and truly 'blooded', there was a return to some kind of 'normality', if one can use that term for such a town as Liverpool then was.

Shortly after the ending of the first epidemic Duncan had written 'fever prevails at all times to a greater or lesser extent among the poor of Liverpool and must continue to prevail so long as their habitations are constructed so as to accumulate filth and to exclude the air of heaven.'

The appalling housing conditions prevailing in the poorer parts of the town were his biggest problem. And the worst features of these were the cellar-dwellings for which Liverpool had become notorious. In fact, the use of cellars as habitations had been banned by law in 1842. Nevertheless in 1847 Duncan found there were still about 30,000 people living in 8000 of these underground, unlit, unventilated quarters.

While still coping with the epidemic, indeed, as part of his plan of action, Duncan launched a massive programme of clearance of the cellars. At the outset these evictions caused great hardship to these unfortunate people, large numbers of whom were left standing in the street. So within a short time, Duncan re-phased the programme so that not more than 100 cellars were cleared in a month, thus giving some opportunity for the people to find somewhere else to go.

Duncan reported on the reluctance of the inmates to leave their miserable abodes because of the facilities offered by the entrances to the cellars 'for the sale of cakes, fruit, vegetables and chips!'. Duncan continued 'and so strong is the feeling that were it not for constant and systematic inspection, the cellars would be re-occupied as soon as they were cleared'.

After three years of determined effort Duncan succeeded in reducing the proportion of people in these down-town areas who were living in cellars from 12 per cent to 2 per cent. No small achievement this, but won at no little social cost.

The relationships between Duncan and his authorities were not always easy and, at times, he must have been glad of the measure of independence attaching to his post. The Select Vestry proved to be particularly difficult. This body corresponded to the Boards of Guardians elsewhere. It was the Select Vestry, and not the Borough Council, which was responsible for the provision of hospital accommodation for the poor, as well as for the relief of destitution. The Vestry continually resented being called upon to spend money to expand hospital provision by Duncan, who, as MOH, was not directly responsible to them.

The dispute came to a head in 1854 when cholera came again. At first the Vestry flatly refused to admit that there was cholera in the town at all. Then, when the epidemic exploded, they took legal advice and declared that it was outside the province of the Medical Officer of Health to recommend 'curative measures', it was his duty simply to 'inspect and report'. Duncan replied by quoting the clause in the Act which required him to 'point out the most efficacious means for checking and preventing the spread of epidemic disease'. The issue was serious enough to be referred to the General Board of Health in London for a ruling. The Board, advised by Chadwick, found in favour of Duncan. It was a victory for him, but more than that, it established a very important principle for the future, which was to last down to our own day.

Duncan's relations with the Borough Council and its Sanitary Committee were almost invariably good. In general, they were very supportive of all that he tried to do. But we must remember that they had never had an MOH before, so they had some learning to do as well.

It is apparent that in Duncan's early years the Council were by no means open-handed in providing him with assistance nor even in covering his necessary expenses.

When in 1851 the Town Clerk asked the various departmental heads to submit a nominal roll of their staff, Duncan replied, perhaps with a touch of wry humour: 'The following list comprises the whole of the officer in my department paid by the Corporation, William Henry Duncan MD, Medical Officer of Health.'

After four years he was still working alone.

In a letter to the Town Clerk written in the same year, he complained that he had paid out of his own pocket upwards of £20 for assistance in his office and had employed his own servant as a messenger. He went on to point out that he had also used his own gig with his horse and groom at an estimated cost to himself of £90.

These were among the teething problems of the new office. In time the Council provided him with clerical staff, and five lodging-house inspectors. Later still, a Dr Cameron was appointed to act as his deputy.

But they never raised his salary! This had been fixed at £750 in 1848 and there it remained for the next 15 years. Although, let it be said in Liverpool's favour, that this was more than any other MOH in the land was being paid at that time.

The years following the great epidemics saw steady improvements in the living and working conditions in Liverpool, especially in the poorer districts. The worst of the sanitary evils were swept away. Private building was controlled; landlords were no longer allowed to build houses in narrow courts and without proper sanitary facilities. Drainage, water supplies, street cleansing and waste disposal were all improved. These improvements were reflected in measurable improvements in the health of the inhabitants. The mortality rate fell from 36 per 1000 in 1846 to 28 per 1000 in 1860, while the average age at death rose from 19 years in 1846 to 25.5 years in 1860. Such changes in mortality statistics may seem small to us today but they represented the saving of many hundreds of lives in a town with a population of 400,000.

After 1860 Duncan's health began to fail and he died three years later at the age of 57 while still in office.

Throughout the 16 years during which he had held the post of Medical Officer of Health, Duncan had carried out his duties conscientiously and well. In tackling the immense problems which faced him he took sensible, practical action based on his belief in the miasma. If the theory was wrong, the action was right. The citizens of Liverpool had good reason to be grateful for his dedication to the sanitary task which undoubtedly brought them substantial benefits.

But more than this William Henry Duncan was a trail-blazer, who, working very largely single-handed, and with very limited resources, pointed the way along the path of sanitary reform and health improvement which his successors in office were to follow through the remainder of the century and even after.

How can we sum up Duncan, assess his contribution and his place in history? He made no original discoveries; he did not contribute to national policy. In this respect he was overshadowed by his more famous contemporary, John Simon. For whereas Simon moved from the local to the national stage, and played his part there, and did so supremely well; Duncan remained in the local scene, playing his part in that more restricted setting, but doing so there with equal success.

Without in any way intending to be derogatory one can say that he was the local lad who made good. But he made much good; for Liverpool was a much better place for its people to live in as a result of his 16 years of unremitting toil.

But what was his legacy? As we have seen he has one distinction which cannot be taken away, he was the first man in. His was the first foot-print in the sand and in this he left an enduring mark.

When five years after his death Alexander Stewart carried out a sanitary survey in the towns of England, he found that many large towns including Manchester, Birmingham and Sheffield had not even bothered to appoint an MOH, they regarded him as an expensive luxury they could afford to do without. But when he came to Liverpool how different is his report. 'There,' he writes, *'the Officer of Health is not only a reality; he is a power in the commonwealth.* He is recognized by the civic authorities as their official adviser whose opinion is asked for and listened to with deference in all matters relating to the public health, and having proved himself worthy of their confidence, he has been entrusted with very large discretionary powers which he has exercised with great tact and judgement in furtherance of the views of the health committees and the Sanitary Acts'. An eloquent testimony to the groundwork laid by Duncan and his immediate successor William Trench.

But what has all this got to do with us and our concerns today? Has history any light to shed on our present? Let me offer a few tentative thoughts.

Duncan shared with us the belief that prevention is to be preferred to cure, where it makes sense to speak of cure. But where it does not, as with so many of the chronic conditions of today, I think he would have agreed that prevention is better than treatment, especially when that treatment takes us into high and costly medical technology, or involves continuing care perhaps lasting a life-time. The case for prevention remains as strong in our day as in his.

Duncan was well aware of what we now call 'the inequalities in health', indeed, he faced them, and this is a problem that continues to plague us today, as the writings of Professor Morris and others have shown. And indeed, Merseyside still looms large in the ranks of the deprived areas of the country.

Housing, bad housing, with all its evil ramifications, still remains a problem here as elsewhere; and Toxteth, which for Duncan meant a pleasant suburb with a park and a hospital, has come to have other connotations associated not so much with disease as with disorder. But, is the new public health concerned

with these problems; or have we cut ourselves off from our roots? I think
perhaps we have.

William Henry Duncan was a medical sanitarian working in the field of
traditional public health. He was faced with the problems of cholera and the
other fevers. Today's community physician, working in and developing the new
public health, is concerned not with cholera but with coronaries, with cancer,
with chronic conditions and addictions. Duncan's problems stemmed largely
from dirt, deficiency and deprivation, ours largely from excess – from excessive
smoking, eating, drinking, speeding, licence. Duncan's targets were filth and
overcrowding; ours are behaviour and lifestyle.

Duncan tackled his problems through the methods of what we now call
primary prevention, that is, the methods of environmental control. We tackle
ours through health education and the screening programmes and therapies of
secondary and tertiary prevention.

Would that our methods were as certain as his! But let us not be disheartened.
Remember, it took fifty years from Duncan's appointment before the Public
Health movement could look up from its work and say 'Well, that's that, we
have now cleaned up the worst evils of an insanitary environment, cholera and
the fevers have been overcome.' Then, with the turn of the century they took
up the task of creating and developing the personal health services we have
with us today.

We still have some time left before the end of our present century, time in
which, if we are persistent and painstaking in applying the best we know, as
Duncan did, we may yet achieve a breakthrough towards a reduction in the
incidence of the plagues that have affected our society since the war. By which
I mean coronary heart disease, lung cancer, death and disablement on the road,
the large but largely hidden problem of alcoholism, the rising problem of drug
addiction, and the massive problem of unwanted pregnancies.

Time still to break the back of these problems if we buckle to the task. But
time too, I think, to remind ourselves that it is sixty years since Lord Dawson
introduced us to the idea of the Health Centre with his famous dictum that
'Preventive and Curative Medicine cannot be separated on any known principle'.
Time at long last to take that lesson really to heart and through the setting up
of good primary health care centres and services out in the community, to bring
that dictum to reality. Recently, Tudor Hart and others have proposed that the
doctors in these centres should take on the responsibility for the public health
in their neighbourhoods. This might require a new kind of doctor – a practitioner
of curative and preventive medicine and of the wider public health. If it does
mean that, so be it. We created a new kind of doctor here in Liverpool in 1847,
we did it again in 1974, we could do it again by 1994, perhaps even here in
Liverpool. A practitioner of medicine and health? That's a thought! But let me
leave that thought there and return again to Duncan.

When an outbreak of infectious disease occurred in Liverpool, the first that
Duncan knew about it was when he was notified of a death, by which time the

epidemic could have been well under way and it would have been too late to do much about it.

It did not take the medical officers of health long to realize that what they needed was the immediate notification of the first case. So through their collective voice, the Society of Medical Officers of Health, they began to agitate for the compulsory notification of infectious diseases. The general practitioners did not want this. They regarded it as an unwarranted intrusion in their private practice. The Government did not want it either because they feared that it might lead to an increased demand for hospital accommodation. But, undaunted, the MOHs continued their pressure until, in the end, they won the day and got what they asked for. That was the old, the traditional, public health.

Now where is the collective voice of the new public health? Who speaks to Government today about the anti-health factors in our society, about the opposition to fluoridation, or sports sponsorship by tobacco interests or 'inequalities' or the needs of inner cities or of the mentally handicapped or the elderly? Have we handed over our responsibilities to ASH, to the Child Poverty Action Group, to SHELTER, to MIND and to Age Concern? And if so, for what benefit? Was it just to achieve a tidy system of administration for the Health Service?

Duncan and his successors developed and practised what became the characteristic, the traditional, roles of the MOH. He was at once public watchdog and accuser, he was adviser and initiator, he was educator and protector.

Now who exercises these roles today? The Environmental Health Officer perhaps. Dr Duncan never passed his responsibilities over to Mr Fresh. But perhaps we do not need them any more. Are our roles as manager, monitor and manipulator of resources enough? I wonder.

Forty years ago, William Beveridge spoke of the five giants which would assail our society after the war. They were Ignorance, Idleness, Squalor, Want and Disease. These giants did not first see the light of day in 1945. Duncan knew them well enough here in Liverpool in 1845 and we do not have to look far to find them here still. They remain a continuing challenge to all those who are concerned with the well-being of the people of this City and this country, and not least, to those who are practitioners of *community health* in its widest sense. Can we lift our eyes from our desks to meet it? I think we can – I think we should.

Finally, next year, the Community Physician will reach the age of ten. He will no longer be a toddler, he will have found his feet. In six years time, in 1990, he will have served the community at large for as long as Duncan did his, here in Liverpool.

Would that some scribe will write of him then; as he once wrote of Duncan, '*He is not only a reality; he is a power in the commonwealth*'.

Acknowledgements

I would like to record my thanks to Professor R Shields, Dean of the Faculty of Medicine, and Dr J.R. Ashton of the department of Community Health in the University of Liverpool who were responsible for arranging the lecture; to my colleagues in the department of Community Health at the London School of Hygiene and Tropical Medicine for their helpful comments; to Miss J Smith, Liverpool City Archivist for her assistance; and to Miss Beth Shaw for clerical help.

The Health Education Council generously provided support for the lecture.

Bibliography

Bradford Hill, A. (1937) *Principles of Medical Statistics,* 1st edn, Lancet, London.

Brockington, C.F. (1965) *Public Health in the Nineteenth Century.* London, Livingstone.

Chave, S.P.W. (1980) The Rise and Fall of the Medical Officer of Health. *Community Health* 2, 36.

Duncan, W.H. (1844) *The Physical Causes of the High Rate of Mortality in Liverpool.* Liverpool.

Duncan, W.H. *The Letter Books (1849–1863)* 3 vols. unpublished MSS. in Liverpool City Archives.

Duncan, W.H. *Report to the Health Committee on the Health of the Town* during the years 1847–48–49–50 then annually 1851 to 1860. Liverpool. Harris.

Finer S.E. (1952) *The Life and Times of Sir Edwin Chadwick* London, Methuen.

Finn M.W. (ed.) (1964) *Report on the Sanitary Condition of the Labouring Population of Great Britain* Chadwick E. (1842) University Press Edinburgh.

Frazer W.H. (1947) *Duncan of Liverpool.* London, Hamish Hamilton.

Frazer W.M. (1950) *A History of English Public Health, 1839–1939.* London, Balliere, Tindall and Cox.

Hope E.W. (1931) *Health at the Gateway.* Cambridge University Press.

Hyde F.E. (1971) *Liverpool and the Mersey.* Newton Abbot, David and Charles.

Interdepartmental Committee on Social Insurance and Allied Services Report. (1942) (Beveridge Report) HMSO, London.

Lambert R. (1963) *Sir John Simon, 1816–1904 and English Social Administration.* London, MacGibban and Kee.

Lewis R.A. (1952) *Edwin Chadwick and the Public Health Movement, 1832–1854.* London, Longmans.

Liverpool Sanitary Act, 1846. Vic. 9 and 10, Cap 127, CXXII.

Midwinter E.C. (1971) *Old Liverpool.* Newton Abbot, David and Charles.

Ministry of Health, Consultative Council on Medical and Allied Services (1920) Interim Report on the Future Provision of Medical and Allied Services (Dawson Report). HMSO. London.

Morris J.N. (1969) Tomorrow's Community Physician. *Lancet* 2, 811.

Morris J.N. (1979) Social inequalities undiminished. *Lancet* 1, 87.

Muir J.R.B. (1907) *A History of Liverpool.* London, Williams and Norgate.

Poor Law Commission (1842) Reports on the Sanitary Condition of Local Populations of England, No.19 Liverpool, HMSO London.

Public Health (1905) Jubilee Number. Chapters 3–5.

Punch (1847) The Value of Health in Liverpool 12, 44.

Royal Commission for inquiring into the State of Large towns and Populous Districts. First Report, 184 (Chairman, Duke of Buccleuth): Section on 'Special

Reports on the Sanitary Condition of Several Towns No. 1. Liverpool. London, HMSO.

Simon J. (1890) *English Sanitary Institutions*. London, Cassell.

Stewart A. (1867) *The Medical and Legal Aspects of Sanitary Reform*. London, Hardwicke.

Townsend P. (ed.) (1982) *Inequalities in Health (Black Report)* Harmondsworth, Middlesex.

Tudor Hart J. (1981) A new kind of doctor. *J. Roy. Soc. Med.* 74, 871.

Requests for reprints to: Dr S. P. W. Chave, Department of Community Health, London School of Hygiene and Tropical Medicine, Keppel Street, London WC1E 7HT.

Medical Officers of Health and Health Services

G. E. Godber. *Community Medicine*, © Oxford University Press, 1986, Vol. 8, No. 1, pp. 1–14.

Introduction

In 1983 I decided to end an already over-long career of speaking and writing about health care. I am breaking that self-imposed silence today for two reasons. Firstly I was asked to speak on an historical subject with which I was more closely involved, over the half century on which I shall reminisce, than anyone who is not a surviving Medical Officer of Health. I can therefore pay a dispassionate tribute to a group of public servants who have not received the credit they deserve. Secondly I have recently read some sadly misinformed academic views on the same subject. I hope I can put the record straight from personal experience but in relation to people and not statistics of services.

It happened that I was close to an older generation, being an honorary member of both the county borough group of MOsH and the County Medical Officers Association 35 years ago. So the generation of MOsH I got to know, then and earlier, during World War II while running a Region for the Ministry, was the post World War I group, most of whom had war experience and came into Public Health at a time when it was moving on from the sanitary revolution of the previous half century to the development of personal health service. The school medical service, as it was then called, had been planned by George Newman, a former MOH, who in 1920, assumed the wider responsibilities of Chief Medical Officer of the new Ministry of Health as well as of the Board of Education where he had been for some time. Maternity and Child Welfare, formerly voluntary and patchy, had become a duty of larger Local Authorities. Clinical services for Tuberculosis and Venereal Diseases were also a duty and were being rapidly developed. Midwives and Nursing Homes were under the MOH's supervision and half way through the inter-war period, reforms long overdue in the Poor Law brought him more and more into the planning and development of hospital services. The old sanitary responsibilities were still there; designation of unfit houses still had to be done by the MOH, but the Public Health Inspectorate (then still called 'Sanitary Inspector') was developing on lines which were to make it independent after 1974. Medical pioneering in sanitary science was largely over, which was just as well because the energies of the MOH were more and more required for co-ordination and development of clinical services and for a new range of preventive activities especially immunisation, which were basically medical, as sanitary science is not. It may be a medical job to set standards of potability for water at least partly – but remedial action is for engineers.

If this all seems ancient history, it does seem to me necessary to show how and why we moved towards a health service for the nation, in order to explain why it was set up, in the way and at the time it was. The Dawson Report which (in 1920) envisaged an integrated service, organised regionally, was not implemented, but it was the 'ghost in the machine' for the next 20 years. More or less consciously the services of local authorities were guided by the MOsH in the direction suggested by the Dawson Committee.

Development of services in major authorities

There were more than 150 MOsH of major authorities and I do not claim to have known them all equally. Therefore when I now quote the work of individuals whom I did know, they are representative of many others. London County was even more atypical then than now, and most of my examples come from elsewhere. Birmingham under H. P. Newsholme, is a good example with fewer problems than more northerly cities. Matthew Burn, Newsholme's deputy and successor, promoted the highly successful general hospitals at Dudley Road and Selly Oak, in which the first successful demonstration of anti-bacterial drugs in the treatment of lobar pneumonia was undertaken by Wilfrid Gaisford, later Professor of Paediatrics in Manchester. Ethel Cassie followed by Jean Mackintosh developed Maternity and Child Welfare work and, at Sorrento Maternity Hospital under Victoria (Mary) Crosse, the first special baby care unit in the country. It is surprising that Birmingham was one of the last authorities to make the MOH also Principal School Medical Officer. Nearby Wolverhampton, like the West Riding of Yorkshire, insisted on keeping its institutions under Public Assistance. Tate with his deputy and successor Macauley in Middlesex and Ferguson with his deputy, Patterson in Surrey built up high quality general hospital services in outer London areas of rapidly growing population where voluntary hospitals could not keep pace. John Charles, later to be Chief Medical Officer, planned developments at the Newcastle General Hospital – notably in neurosurgery, radiotherapy and pae-diatrics, development with which the Newcastle city hospitals could not keep pace. Sheffield's hospital services owed a great deal to Sir James Clarke, the Medical Superintendent of the City General Hospital for 40 years. He was there as the Resident Medical Officer in the Poor Law Institution in 1912 but worked closely with Rennie the MOH, whose deputy he was. Leeds under Johnston Jarvis, Bradford under J. J. Buchan, Hull under Gebbie, Bristol under Parry, W. M. Frazer in Liverpool and Veitch Clark in Manchester and Nottingham, Derby and Leicester under Banks, Lilico and Macdonald respectively, all made great advances in the 1930s. Other counties had less opportunity but Lindsey under Campbell and Lancashire under first Butterworth and then Hall made progress. Some of the county tuberculosis services, especially Lancashire's guided by Lissant-Cox and Nottinghamshire's by Tibbits, were notable examples.

London was a special problem, but under Menzies and later Allen Daley it had made considerable progress in providing better services in a larger number of old general hospitals especially in obstetrics. The Royal Postgraduate Medical School at Hammersmith Hospital was formerly a London County Council hospital, and it required great foresight and pertinacity, particularly from Daley, to get the school established. The most important message from the Dawson report was that a regional organisation was essential and although Middlesex, Surrey and the LCC might have had some semblance of integrated services, they were not what was required.

The clearest positive move towards regions could have come from The Cancer Act, 1939 but it came too late to be given effect before the war. This act made it a duty of Local Authorities to make arrangements for the diagnosis and treatment of cases of cancer. It was expected that a number of authorities in a region would base arrangements on one appropriate hospital. Only Lincolnshire achieved a scheme and that was a smaller unit than was intended. I was with Ernest Brown, then Minister of Health, when he opened the new centre at the Scunthorpe Memorial Hospital. It was quite a nice little centre but in the wrong place. There were also one or two initial snags about it. The day before he arrived to open it they found that they had not put in an electricity main which was rather essential for radiotherapy. The architect had planned a fine new system for a light lock in the diagnostic radiological department – a revolving door – but he had not measured the Sister-in-Charge and she got stuck with the door half way round on the morning before Ernest Brown arrived!

Maternal and child health

Between the wars, services for mothers, babies and school children were much improved through the activities of Public Health Departments though with some friction with the general practitioners and not a great deal of help from the paediatric and obstetric hospitals. Nevertheless, the first chair of Child Health was set up in Newcastle, again during World War II, based on the City General Hospital and occupied by James Spence. The chair at Great Ormond Street, usually regarded as the premier centre of paediatrics, came later. The first obstetrician established in Lincolnshire was appointed by the County Council which, like the West Riding, had built modern maternity homes. McKeown's followers will say that the steady fall in infant mortality was due to better mother care and nutrition and not to technical medical or allied services. That may be partly, but not wholly true, and the educational work of health visitors and medical officers was the main reason for both. M'Gonigle's work on nutrition in Stockton-on-Tees showed all too clearly how ill nourished the poorest still were. Jean Mackintosh of Birmingham, the first woman ever to be President of the Society of MOsH, was the exemplar. There were many others, long before hospital-based obstetricians and paediatricians generally accepted their responsibilities for prevention. Yet Leonard Parsons the first Professor of Children's Diseases in Birmingham set the tone for them in the first post-war Blair-Bell Lecture to the RCOG on 'Antenatal Paediatrics'.[1] The School Health Service was also an important factor in promoting the health of children. If the BPA and the RCOG are now leaders in this field they got their impulse from Public Health. The report of the House of Commons Committee[2] is good evidence that they have at last learnt the lesson. When I took the DPH in 1936 it was a statutory requirement for a MOH, but after that, one had to spend at least a year or two doing routine clinic work with school children and mothers and babies in a way far less constructive than preventive paediatrics is today. It did, however, give a period for re-orientation from the nine months course in which so much time was spent on sanitary law and bacteriology and chemistry of water and milk. The memory of that kind of routine may well explain the ambivalence so many clinicians still show towards Public Health even in its later form of Community Medicine.

World War II

The strength of Public Health Departments and the personal authority of the MOsH were essential to the organisation of the emergency services for Civil Defence in World War II. They ran the First Aid services, improvised an ambulance service using, perforce, vehicles which would horrify the ambulance staff of today and were the agents through whom the Ministry of Health's Hospital Officers for Regions controlled the hospital arrangements for casualties. Even in rural areas, which received literally millions of women and children evacuated from the City Centres and the south coast, MOsH were heavily engaged in arranging services. In the North Midlands alone, 500 maternity beds were improvised in country mansions and the like with a remarkable record of safety over five years of operation. There were innumerable instances of MOsH playing key roles in civil defence, but two will suffice.

Arthur Massie had to handle the casualty services of Coventry in the first saturation raid on a provincial city, and that included all the health problems of disrupted water supply and sewage disposal as well as the casualty service. Stanley Walton, later to be Professor at the London School of Hygiene was awarded the George Medal for his personal behaviour when West Bromwich, of which he was the MOH, was attacked.

Infectious diseases

The traditional responsibilities for control of infectious disease became especially important, not only when water, sewage and cleansing services were interrupted, but also as a result of population movement and the crowding which occurred in air raid shelters. An extreme example was in Glasgow in 1942 when a group of Poles returning from the Middle East brought smallpox with them. Alexander Macgregor and his deputy Robert Peters, were mainly responsible for the control of that outbreak. The patients were all admitted to an isolation hospital at

Robroyston and no one could understand how one case of smallpox had happened to occur in a long-stay resident (an elderly man) in a hospital at the other side of the city. At least no one overtly understood but there were people behind the scenes who knew that one of the staff at the mental hospital had a regular assignation with one of the staff in the grounds of Robroyston. Small things are concealed at the time of the smallpox epidemics. Perhaps we were lucky to escape a major influenza epidemic for so long (if one discounts a smaller episode in 1943) but Liverpool in 1951 nearly experienced a serious epidemic of influenza – not in mortality but in the number of severe cases. By then diphtheria, which formerly affected 50,000 children a year, had been controlled by immunisation. It may be a justified criticism that immunisation should have been used effectively much earlier, as it was in Canada, but none the less from the end of 1941 and despite Civil Defence burdens and shortage of staff, MOsH ran such an effective campaign that deaths were down by a third within a year and both incidence and mortality were down by three quarters by 1946. There has been nothing else like it and even Tom McKeown cannot brush that one aside. For the last 35 years diphtheria has been so rare a disease that it is likely to be missed, since few doctors have seen a single case, yet 45 years ago there would always have been patients in the wards of infectious diseases hospitals such as Fazakerley.

The disease could and should have been eradicated much earlier, but until the NHS Act of 1946 there was, in fact, no explicit statutory authority for immunisation, except against smallpox. Until then we were using a 50-year-old provision which allowed councils of Districts to provide 'medicines' for the 'poorer members of the population'. It is wonderful what you can do by a bit of quick interpretation. In retrospect it seems extraordinary that Parliament made no provision in the Public Health Act of 1936, perhaps an early example of Governments' disregard of health promotion. The Public Health laboratory Service was used to supply the antigens and the Ministry undertook central publicity, but the real outcome depended on the energy of the local MOH and none failed, if some were 'more equal than others'.

Treatment programmes for what were then called venereal diseases had been organised by MOsH for 20 years and the incidence was declining at the beginning of the War, but the wartime disturbance of ordinary family life produced an increase as it had in 1914–1918. This time MOsH were better prepared and managed to keep some control, through far better organised tracing of contacts and the temporary requirements of notification. John Charles in Newcastle was one of the pioneers of better contact tracing, based on clinics, and it says something for the preventative system that the increase in these diseases in recent years, large as it is, has been less here than in most other countries except China.

Beginnings of the NHS

Altogether the part played by MOsH of counties and cities in the improvement of health care between 1920 and 1946 might reasonably have led them to expect a different role from the one they were given in the NHS. The original White Paper on the NHS in 1944 envisaged a system in which counties and county boroughs would still have owned and run their hospitals and those of the county districts too in all probability, and they would also have had a co-ordinating role with the other hospitals. Had that happened, the service would have been ill co-ordinated because of local competition between hospitals and there would have been no effective regional control. It was Bevan's contribution to the Act that cut through the hesitancy and established a regionally-planned and locally-managed hospital service unimpeded by local government boundaries. Hospital Management Committees could operate their groups for the benefit of the whole population of a district in the way the wartime hospital surveys had clearly shown was needed. Regional Boards were able to plan and develop specialist services taking a broader than local view. Two leading MOsH, Veitch Clark of Manchester and Topping, Daley's deputy in London, had been among the Surveyors, all of whom reached the same view on those principles.

The Senior Administrative Medical Officers of the new Regional Hospital Boards played key roles in the early years of the NHS and outstanding among them were the MOsH Macaulay of Middlesex, Patterson of Surrey, Williams of Oxford and the Liverpool SAMO Trevor Lloyd Hughes. Ewen of East Anglia and Davies soon to succeed Williams, were also from Middlesex and Williamson returned to Leeds from Portsmouth. Public health therefore contributed important leadership in the hospital development, but that was a digression from the mainstream of prevention and health promotion for which MOsH were primarily trained. Most senior MOsH remained with their Councils and it is with their contribution to the NHS in that traditional role that I am mainly concerned. Hospital services were inevitably, and for years increasingly, the most costly part of the NHS. That is not wrong; the care of the sick must cost more when they are most sick and most dependent. Prevention is not an alternative, because death is not indefinitely preventable. We all have to die and most of us will be sick and dependent in a terminal period, even if it is mercifully short and prevention has to be aimed at reducing that. But we have learned in the NHS, and practised more than most countries that less expensive care outside hospitals is to be preferred to care within them, so long as it is equally effective in human terms; the great contribution of the MOsH to the NHS was their organisation of support and preventive services related to health care. Some of them like George Gibson of Leicestershire and Fred Hall of Lancashire also made notable contributions as members of Regional Boards, but most played other, too little recognised but most effective, parts at the local level in HMCs or Executive Councils.

Local Health Authorities were required by the 1946 Act not only to prepare schemes for their own services but also to consult hospital authorities and the Executive Councils running the practitioner services. The LHAs therefore had a key role in the first attempt to develop a comprehensive national programme for preventive and support services. Some of the services were new to LHAs, some long familiar, and some, like the ambulance service, linked to wartime experience. Most of the programme was obligatory, but some like home help services were optional, though all provided them. One of my jobs at the Ministry in 1947 was to read all those schemes (142 of them) and try to make certain that none were either unusually meagre or exceptionally extravagant. There were very few extravagances and just the odd case of obvious inadequacy. The main point was to make sure that schemes were not so specific as to tie up the authorities in strait jackets for the future. Together, those schemes provided the outline of the most extensive support system in any country I know. Their value and success deserve more recognition than they had.

The NHS does not stand isolated; it is part of the caring base of our society which extends from cash supports under National Insurance through assisted housing, education and social welfare to technical, medical and allied care of the most sophisticated kind. It uses what the French call the social budget which is a little more than half our national budget, and its integration makes it the least expensive in the western world. Admittedly our level of social support is too low and the incomes of the health profession are lower than in other countries either in absolute or relative terms, but we derive more from what we do spend: something of which our politicians too often seem lamentably ignorant. MOsH have not been given enough credit for their part in securing the needed integration.

Now that community nursing services have been re-grouped under nursing leadership, it is easily forgotten that the reorganisation which brought that about was effected under the leadership of County and County Borough MOsH. Home Help services were first established by Health Departments over twenty years before they were, quite properly, handed over to social services departments. Ambulance services were mostly developed from the wartime systems even though voluntary agencies played a part: only in Scotland were they organised otherwise. MOsH lost their direct administrative responsibility for hospitals, and some of them, especially some of the older ones, bitterly resented that after contributing so much to progress in the 30s. In the main they applied themselves effectively to the preventive and supportive role and in so doing came closer to their original and distinctive function than would have been possible otherwise.

The novelty and scale of the reorganisation of hospital and specialist services have obscured the extent of the progress Local Authorities made. Yet this should be seen in retrospect as under-pinning the whole of the NHS. By the 1960s it had become the common medical rhetoric to condemn the 'tripartite' administration of the NHS and nowhere more stridently than in the profession's own Porritt Report. I have never subscribed to that. There were three components each with its own problems of change and advance. It would have been a calamity if the family practitioner and preventive services had been subordinated and largely forgotten by new authorities overwhelmed by the size and complexity of hospital and specialist problems. It is worth noting that New Zealand, which established its own Health Service eight years before ours, has only started to bring management of the other services under the same elected boards as the hospitals within the last year. There certainly was a problem of coordination which was met more effectively through the goodwill and understanding of progressive MOsH than by any other means. London had a special problem with the four Metropolitan Regions and the county MO. Sir Allen Daley, organised liaison meetings of the MOsH and SAMOs which I often attended in the early days, just as provincial SAMOs did for their Regions. Reorganisation had to come in 1974 if only because the long overdue reorganisation of Local Government occurred then, and again in 1982 to correct some of the mistakes made in 1974, but the preceding years had been highly productive.

Prevention of disease

I propose now to pick out some of the individual contributions to services which were unobtrusive and so have had little recognition. Prevention of communicable disease was the chief original function of the MOH and it was mainly achieved through the sanitary revolution. The problems were changing because better nutrition and a better environment not only reduced the liability of children to meet some infections, but also made them better able to tolerate universal diseases like measles and whooping cough which formerly had killed many hundreds every year. Even as late as the early 1930s some 800 children out of every 100,000 died of the common notifiable infective diseases of childhood every year; that number is now six or less. Diphtheria was virtually eliminated by immunisation and cases of whooping cough greatly reduced. After a field trial conducted by the MRC through MOsH, poliomyelitis vaccine was used generally and by 1963 the incidence was reduced by 90 per cent and has since been minimal. The public was not easily persuaded until the sad death of a brilliant young footballer made people suddenly conscious of the risk their children ran. Alec Hutchison as MOH of Hull was able to halt one of our last local outbreaks by a three-day immunisation campaign in 1961. Tetanus was reduced to a very low level by the adoption of a combined vaccine: measles and rubella vaccine and BCG for school leavers complete the present programme but there may well be more to follow. Anthrax vaccine was required only for those specially exposed at work and yellow fever and cholera vaccines only for travellers.

In all this programme of immunisation MOsH played the essential local part, but the strategy has to be national. High levels of protection can only be obtained through local tactical handling. Some MOsH like John Warin of Oxford, were able to achieve a very high level of success through use of their close relationship with general practitioners. Tom Galloway of West Sussex was the pioneer of the computer-based system which is now widely used. Success could have been much more complete if the government had been prepared to push in the way those of New Zealand, the Netherlands and the USA have done. Without that, the split responsibility coupled with a good deal of ambivalence among doctors and some misguided propaganda by a few medical antagonists have left us with far too low a level of immunisation against measles and whooping cough and a smaller but dangerous shortfall against some other infections.

The Public Health Laboratory Service evolved from the wartime emergency service and it has made control of infections and field investigation much easier. MOsH still occasionally faced local outbreaks in which they had to use all the traditional skills of their predecessors. The last large typhoid epidemic occurred in Aberdeen in the spring of 1965, the result of contamination of corned beef sold from a shop in which one infected can was opened and sliced on a bench where many others were then opened. That incident was only elucidated by Ian MacQueen and his staff because in the previous year three small local outbreaks in England had been shown to be due to macroscopically undetected infection of single cans. Three MOsH in different parts of England each found proof of the infection and the PHLS was able to show how a minute single-strain infection of a can's contents could occur during the cooling process without spoilage of the meat or 'blowing' of the can. Another MOH in North Yorkshire two years earlier had proved infection of canned ham. Looking back into the Ministry records we were able to identify other outbreaks even 40 years earlier in which the same cause could be deduced, yet I was met at first with frank disbelief of this proposition among European colleagues at a WHO meeting when I expounded it. The alertness of those four men made it possible for us to close another loophole in the control of imported food, and one of them a few years later detected the cause of another outbreak, this time due to an accidental chemical contamination during transport of flour with a toxic substance which survived the baking process, and the diagnosis of the clinical cases was poliomyelitis until the original offending chemical was found. There was, and there still is for his successor, a role for the MOH in handling such situations.

There was a very unusual incident in the North Riding a dozen years ago when a village water supply was infected and both human and bovine infection with typhoid followed but the infected milk all went to a distant dairy and was pasteurised before sale and infected no one. It was a real test of epidemiological acumen for the MOH.

The extreme emergency of a smallpox outbreak can no longer occur, since there are now only two carefully guarded laboratory frozen cultures of the variola virus but the last two occurrences of smallpox in Britain followed leakage from research laboratories. The speed and effectiveness of the intervention of Leslie Millar of Birmingham working with his colleagues in the West Midlands brought the last incident rapidly under control. Before the WHO Smallpox Eradication Campaign, the disease was imported at irregular intervals, especially after air travel became the rule. In 1961/62 during a period of unusually large immigration from the Indian sub-continent, six separate importations occurred and were quickly contained. I remember particularly John Douglas of Bradford handling an extraordinary incident in which the index case, a child with malaria, and the two second generation cases were all dead without having developed focal rashes before the first identifiable skin rash appeared in a third generation case. You all have very good reason to be grateful to WHO for having, since 1972, protected us finally from smallpox, and also from the complications and expense of primary vaccination.

There are still outbreaks of food-borne infection from time to time, most commonly of the communal kitchen type as occurred recently in a Yorkshire hospital but water and milk have been made reasonably safe and community-wide infections are now usually due to respiratory spread. There is not yet a reliable means of controlling epidemic influenza. Tuberculosis is still a problem although it is now small. The anti-tuberculosis drugs have been used with such effect that most of us have forgotten that this disease was called with some truth, as well as Edwardian grandiloquence 'captain of the men of death'. Tuberculosis caused almost 47,000 new cases and over 24,000 deaths as recently as 1944 in England and Wales alone. The new drugs not only made pulmonary tuberculosis usually curable and meningitis often so: they also made patients non-infectious quickly. That meant that primary infection in childhood protecting many but leaving others liable to breakdown and disease in adolescence or early adult life, soon became an uncommon event. MOsH were able to give protection to exposed and to older children with BCG vaccine and to use mass radiography for detection of pulmonary infection in adults. As mass campaigns became relatively unproductive they could use the technique provided by Hospital Board teams more selectively and as a diagnostic resource for GPs. Some cities still had major problems in the late '50s, especially in Scotland. Kenneth Cowan had moved from Essex to Scotland as CMO and it was on his initiative that the miniature radiographic resources of the whole country were mobilised for special campaigns, first in Glasgow and later in the other Scottish cities to try to find the unknown and infective sufferers from tuberculosis. Later Andrew Semple in Liverpool set up a more successful campaign using the same resources to improve the position of Liverpool after more than 80 per cent of the adult population were screened. Both surveys were needed but here success led to diminished use thereafter. I always regretted our failure to use Andrew Semple's indigenous local voluntary worker to encourage others to take advantage of a valuable preventive programme. The USSR does it with great effect all the time. The first full scale field trial of BCG in any country was organised by the MRC with the help of MOsH and it justified the general use of BCG for school leavers from 1954 on. Just how large a part BCG has played in controlling tuberculosis in the last 30 years must be uncertain. It may well be that the introduction of universal pasteurisation of milk and the eradication programme by the Ministry of Agriculture, Fisheries and Food 10 years earlier was as important.

MOsH used their epidemiological skills in the control of other illnesses. For instance they had done the field work for the maternal deaths enquiry started in 1936 and remained the initiators of the process in the new confidential enquiry which began in 1952 and is still running. Retrolental fibroplasia, causing blindness in premature babies was shown to be associated with the use of high concentrations of oxygen in incubators in a study carried out locally by MOsH but coordinated centrally by Katherine Hirst. The effect of maternal rubella on the foetus was shown in another study coordinated by Margaret Manson. The study of infant mortality has been facilitated by MOsH collating information on birth weights. The enquiry into the thalidomide disaster and the subsequent recording of congenital abnormalities again required local action by MOsH. The prototype perinatal mortality studies reported by Frank Riley were joint efforts of MOsH, paediatricians and obstetricians in three areas and have been more widely used since. Alison MacFarlane's editorial[3] in the BMJ pointed the way to future advance. There was and is no alternative to the coordinating activity of the MOH or his successor the Community Physician in this way.

Fluoridation of water is the classic example of another kind of health promotion in which MOsH would lead if the politicians would let them. Gwilym Wynne Griffith in Anglesey skilfully managed his own authority and public opinion in the county to secure fluoridation in the first test period. He had an ingenious method of dealing with people who would complain. The start of the scheme was announced for a particular day and the next week they collected the usual flood of complaints about the taste in the water and then they let out the news that the start had been postponed for a week. He was later to pilot a UK resolution through the 20th World Health Assembly in favour of fluoridation. Leslie Millar persuaded Birmingham, bringing in the largest number of beneficiaries in the country, a decade later. Most MOsH have experienced the frustration of failing to persuade local councillors and members of water authorities to face the legal uncertainties and undertake one of the simplest health promotion initiatives still remaining. Successive ministers and governments have feebly failed to legislate on lines their counterparts in New Zealand and the Irish Republic have successfully used. This is the classic example of political ambivalence about health promotion: ministers always want to be seen to favour prevention and be on the side of the good even if only because it may save cost but they will not run the risk of losing a few votes. As one said to me, 'There's no political mileage in that'.

Now that the problems of early acute infection are so much reduced the epidemiology of congenital abnormalities and chronic disease has become more important and more amenable to intervention. Screening for unapparent abnormalities was a large part of maternity, child welfare and school health service work. Now there is a wider range of detectable disease or handicap conditions – testing the neonate for hypothyroidism or congenital hip disease or Down's Syndrome, for example. Screening for unapparent handicap is still important, deafness, visual and orthopaedic defects for example but different processes are used for adults. Multiphasic screening is no longer the vogue, even in North America, and we were spared excesses here because of critical evaluation. The real future for screening lies with general practice, but the MOsH have had their part in its rational promotion and they will have to go on in that part in association with primary care in the future.

A whole range of new uncertainties about the effects of chemical or radiation factors in the environment, each with its own critics, has to be assessed. A parliamentary committee has reviewed neonatal mortality[2] but paid too little attention to the community work that has so much reduced it. Family planning has been promoted in the last 20 years and MacGregor in Southampton led the way in taking the service to the homes where it was most needed. I shepherded through the resolution in WHO which got them to play a part, in three weeks UNICEF had followed and in three months the United Nations had set up an international agency (United Nations Fund for Population Activities).

New patterns of care

So far I have talked about the traditional roles of the MOH which are still relevant within the NHS, but the NHS brought new opportunities for MOsH who could use their control of supporting services to promote a better pattern of health care. The clearest opportunity was that of regrouping community services around general practice.

The prototype group practices in Skipton and Dartford did not have health visitors and home nurses working with them, nor did the first health centres. I first saw the advantages when on a WHO Fellowship to Scandinavia in 1954 and spoke of it to the County Borough MOH Group a few weeks later. In the same year two groups in Winchester persuaded Ivor MacDougall of Hampshire to support them by associating health visitors with their work. A little later still John Warin told me that he was developing a similar scheme in Oxford. Others were slow to follow but Warin and MacDougall persisted, with growing support from practitioners and nurses, until suddenly in the early 1960s there was a fairly gentle change of heart. By 1966 Oxford had all its health visitors working in association with general practices. Some leading nurses had opposed the change, and some still do, partly because they fear and may have actually suffered medical attempts to subordinate them. Nevertheless by the late 1960s the majority of practices and of community nurses took part. Despite a recent backlash among health visitors and the shortcomings of some inner city practices the system must be here to stay and it is a major advance, if the kind of organisation Marsh and Kaim-Caudle have described is developed.

Confinement at home is now infrequent but much ante- and post-natal care is undertaken by midwives who also work with group practices. Early discharge after delivery is now common and after care is essential. Very short stay was pioneered in Bradford by Theobald the obstetrician and John Douglas the MOH, and they were able to handle the much increased load in the decade to 1964 when the birth rate rose substantially. London had a similar crisis which was handled less promptly but ultimately in the same way. It is an odd reflection that two weeks was once the normal post-natal stay and even the Cranbrook Committee 25 years ago asked for 10 days. The average is now five days.

The development of community services owes much to George Townsend, the outstanding MOH of Buckinghamshire who also controlled the Welfare

Services for the county and used the opportunity to rationalise multiple visiting systems for special purposes. The health visitors, with his encouragement, pioneered the establishment of young mothers' clubs in the county as a partial alternative to the old-style baby clinic. I recall David Donnison agreeing to undertake one of his earliest studies into that system. There were many other examples of such exploratory initiatives.

Kenneth Macdonald of Leicester had set in train one of the earliest studies of one-parent families. The best known and most comprehensive study of child development through into early adult life was that on A Thousand Families in Newcastle Upon Tyne in which Spence's Department of Child Health collaborated with John Charles in the preparation and with his successors, Stanley Walton and Richard Pearson over more than 20 years, and through the tenure of Donald Court, Spence's successor. A little attention to that study might broaden the views of those who think that there can be equality in health care. Equity in health care would not be equality, the worst off would need the most. The two surveys of British births initiated by Neville Butler and sponsored by the National Birthday Trust were only practicable at all, because of the support of MOsH.

Coordination of services

Coordination within the NHS has always been a difficulty and still is. A special committee of the Central Health Services Council produced a report on it in the early years, without much effect. It was largely through the efforts of MOsH at local level that services were coordinated as well as they were. There was usually one senior MOH on each Regional Board but the wider effect was obtained by MOsH working on Hospital Management Committees or with their staffs. Men like Wallace of the Isle of Wight, Elliot of the West Riding, Wofinden of Bristol, Denninson of Newham, Galloway of West Sussex, Parry Jones of Somerset, Gawne of Lancashire, Ludkin of Durham, Cullington of Berkshire and Andrew Semple of Liverpool are just a few of those who contributed much in this way and in York there was Catherine Crane, the only woman MOH of a county Borough. James Grant of Gateshead and John Warin of Oxford rather unusually had also consultant contracts in communicable disease. But there is a broader context of planning for health care in which MOsH led. The New Towns established just after the war had little provision for planning of anything but housing, industry and amenities. Harlow was lucky in having Stephen Taylor as Vice Chairman and he, with the willing help of Kenneth Cowan of Essex, secured Health Centres in each of the neighbourhoods of the New Town. Kenneth also succeeded in getting a Centre for the housing development at Harold Wood. These were the forerunners of Thamesmead and Guy's Hospital Medical School's interest fostered by John Butterfield as Professor of Experimental Medicine and fully developed under Peter Higgins as Professor of General Practice. Ludkin was later to influence planning for Washington New Town, as did the Scottish Home and Health Department for

Cumbernauld and Livingstone. John Reid of Buckinghamshire gave this planning a new dimension at Milton Keynes by covering the whole health care programme, as did Edgar for the large new development planned at Northampton. Planning has since become a more general activity in the NHS as all have realised that community care really means the integration of hospital work with that outside hospital and with the Social Services.

The Society of Medical Officers of Health and the BMA in their evidence to the Seebohm Committee[4] both urged unification under the direction of the MOH. Behind the scenes I tried to persuade the Society that this was a mistake and that Social Work as a discipline must be allowed to evolve in parallel with and not subordinate to medical work. Their evidence probably had the opposite effect of their intention and hardened the views of the Committee against them and I think the Committee was right. They may well have encouraged an adversarial relationship between the departments that could be seen all too often except where the MOH and the Director of Social Services were both broad minded enough to seize the opportunity of working together. Two MOsH, Meredith Davies the deputy in Liverpool and Denninson in Newham became Directors of Social Services.

Health centres

Heath centres were first proposed in the Dawson Report in 1920 and a very different kind of community centre was given the same name by George Scott Williamson and Innes Pearse 10 years later in Peckham. The NHS dreamers and the Act appeared to expect a rash of such centres to break out in 1948 and especially that they would be used by general medical practitioners and dentists. In fact a score or so of former dispensaries for the poor and the GWR Centre at Swindon were taken over in 1948 and then everybody stopped to think what the Centres were to be and do. Some strange sketch plans were produced and soon forgotten – the one I remembered particularly provided for six GPs and various clinics and included no less than 39 water closets after every kind of segregation by sex, profession and other designation. It did seem an expensive way to provide a public convenience. Edinburgh and London each built one expensive centre, Sighthill and Woodberry Down respectively, for new housing developments. Sheffield adapted some premises which the doctors then declined to use because their colleagues claimed they would have unfair advantages. The simple fact was that doctors were suspicious of 'Town Hall control', the financial arrangements were unfavourable for them and the Councils, and the best pattern of grouping community services had not yet emerged. Once group medical practice had become the norm with community nursing and midwifery staff linked with the practices, the fair financial arrangements negotiated for GPs in the mid sixties gave MOsH the chance to develop. Robert Parry and Robert Wofinden had shown the way with the William Budd Centre in Bristol – the first purpose-built NHS centre to be opened in Britain, and Berkshire with Huddy's guidance and Jeffrey Williams' help had cooperated to convert the Faringdon Cottage Hospital with RHB support into the first newly opened health centre in Britain. Wherever MOsH had been able to secure the interest of their GP colleagues health centres began to appear in considerable numbers from 1964 on. Only 17 centres had been opened in the first 15 years of the NHS but in each ensuing year the number of openings rose rapidly until it reached 100 a year in England alone by the 1970s. Many of the medium-sized authorities such as Bolton were able to move quickly, as were those like Oxford and Hampshire with well-established group practices of doctors with nurses. Ronald Elliot of the West Riding and Joe Lyons in Devonshire managed to persuade their GPs to join in many smaller centres in rural areas as well as centres in town like Castleford where all the GPs joined in. Parry Jones at Frome and MacDougall at Hythe arranged whole town groupings on sites linked with the local hospital. Paddy Donaldson on Teeside even organised one for 26 GPs at premises linked with the bus centre for the district as was also done at Stroud in Gloucestershire. It is a great pity that the great impetus was slowed for political reasons five years ago, and especially that the needs of city centres have not been met as the Acheson report showed.[5]

Changes

It has been characteristic of the evolution of public health in Britain that MOsH would show the way on protection of water supplies, disposal of human wastes, condemnation and replacement of unfit housing, organisation of antenatal care and preventive paediatrics. Then, having proved their point, they would pass on to others technically equipped and qualified, the full development of the programme. The same kind of change has occurred in the NHS. Domestic help for the sick or handicapped in the home was developed by MOsH from 1948 and then rightly turned over to the regrouped Social Services. Social worker support for general practice pioneered in Barnstaple, with Nuffield help and at Darbishire House in Manchester with University help also properly came under the new Social Services Department. In Teeside and in Berkshire I was later to open health centres in which the Social Services Department had their own space in the premises for their local staff. Junior training centres for the mentally handicapped were essentially educational in function for a group that Education Authorities ignored as ineducable until pioneering MOsH had shown how mistaken this was. Adult centres developed in a comparable way and were rightly passed on to Social Services. It was MOsH like Tom Peirson of Plymouth, I. G. Davies of Leeds and Stanley Gawne of Lancashire who opened up the prospect.

Management of mental illness has been changed even more radically. Part of the change was facilitated by the new psychotropic drugs, part by the near-eradication of neurosyphilis but the most important change was in public attitudes to the mentally ill and to the mentally handicapped. The activity policy of psychiatrists such as T.P. Rees, at Warlingham Park, Joshua Carse at Worthing, Bierer with the Marlborough Day Hospital and Duncan Macmillan

at Nottingham in unlocking doors, encouraging early discharge and even preventing the need for admission was only possible because MOsH like S. L.
Wright of Croydon helped with community services. Allen Daley, London
County MOH was the first chairman of the standing mental health advisory
committee and he encouraged these developments. I reported on the pioneer
day hospital in Montreal in 1951 which I visited. Perhaps the most significant
developments were the psychiatric units in general hospitals in the Manchester
Region. Pool of Oldham was the forerunner amongst psychiatrists but he was
working with Chalmers Keddie the MOH just as Rees had worked with Wright
in Croydon. Fraser and his successor, Minto, in Cumberland made similar
changes. Naturally, performance varied widely. Some programmes like immunisation were essentially national and needed stong central support from a
nationally-recommended schedule, others were very much a matter of local
initiative. The wide variation in effectiveness was well shown when, in 1963,
Enoch Powell produced his National Health and Welfare Plan the year after
the Hospital Plan. Nevertheless the gibe that the National Health Service was
really a National Sickness Service was undeserved. Health promotion and disease
prevention made far more progress in the first 25 years of the NHS than has
been recognised. If Parliament had had the resolution to provide effective
measures against tobacco use and the growing consumption of alcohol or clear
statutory support for fluoridation, progress would have been greater still. They
were dilatory over action on wearing of seat belts in cars and crash helmets by
motor cyclists; they do not recognise the need for speed control and are
ambivalent over the strict application of limits on drinking and driving. The
great failure since 1950 has been in the control of smoking-related diseases and
that has been central and political, not peripheral and professional. In the end,
it was Burns of Salford who established the first anti-smoking clinic.

Nevertheless there was an important transition to be made from the function
of the MOH developing services to fill gaps on behalf of priority groups,
authorising local authority hospitals and the control of epidemic disease, to that
of the community physician facilitating services provided by others and helping
districts to coordinate those services and review their effectiveness. Some MOsH
were already making the change – I have named some of them and there were
many others. Some health education seems at last to be coming into its own
led by the Health Education Council and Action on Smoking and Health. Some
MOsH felt less secure in a personal role which was less dependent on a familiar
office machine. I wish they had more help in the 50s and 60s from academic
Social Medicine than they did, even after the Hunter Report of 1972. John
Brotherston made an outstanding contribution in Edinburgh before he moved
to be CMO Scotland but the horizons of other schools seemed for long to be
limited to the statutorily required DPH until Jerry Morris went to the London
School of Hygiene and Tropical Medicine.

Finally, I must mention an area in which some leading MOsH made a special
contribution. Central government needs medical advisers and has often recruited
them from among leading MOsH. Everyone knows of the earlier examples,

John Simon, Arthur Newsholme and George Newman as CMOs, John Charles
was MOH of Newcastle when he came in as deputy to Wilson Jameson to help
organise the NHS. Andrew Davidson was County MOH of the North Riding
when he moved to be CMO Scotland and Robert Peters moved to be his
deputy from being deputy in Glasgow. Arthur Massey was the first CMO of
the Ministry of National Insurance, moving from Coventry. Kenneth Cowan's
move from Essex to Scotland has already been mentioned and John Reed moved
there after first joining the DHSS from Buckinghamshire as one of my deputies.
Deputy Arthur Culley, Dick Bevan and Gareth Crompton all moved to the
Welsh Office from Welsh counties. Other experienced MOsH like I. G. Davies,
Peter Minto, Gwilym Wynne Griffith, Terry Baird and Brian Disdsbury moved
to important posts in central government, which would have been lost without
them.

Progress and the future

At the outset I promised only reminiscence and have mentioned many MOsH
by name though only a fraction of the group. I have tried to indicate, by quoting
examples I knew at first hand, the kind of influence for progress MOsH have
been. There could have been many more and I could have found some negative
and critical comment too. I say no more than that in my experience plus has
far outweighed minus. The lineage of the present and future community
physicians is not unworthy of their own or any other speciality. They deserve
more understanding and more general support than their clinical colleagues
often provide. I know among them some of the most progressive and widely-
informed physicians of today – and for that matter some of the least
self-regarding.

This article is an edited version of the text of an address given by Sir George
Godber as the second Duncan Lecture in Liverpool in December, 1984.

References

1. Parsons L. Antenatal Paediatrics. *Obstet Gynaecol* 1946.53 1 16.
2. House of Commons Social Services Committee. Second Report Session.
   1979–80. Perinatal and Neonatal Mortality, 663–1. London: HMSO, 1980.
3. Macfarlane A. Perinatal mortality surveys *Br Med J* 1984. 281 1473 1474.
4. Committee on local authority and allied personal social services. (Seebohm).
   Report Cmnd 3703 London: HMSO. 1968.
5. Study Group Report – Primary Health Care in Inner London. London: London
   Health Planning Consortium. 1981.

Health for All and Primary Health Care in Europe

Public Health (1987). 101, 151–157, Hakan Hellberg, Director, Department of Public Information and Education for Health, World Health Organisation, 1211 Geneva, Switzerland, © The Society of Community Medicine, 1987.

Introduction

It is now 140 years since the Parliament at Westminster passed the Liverpool Sanitary Act and 139 years since William Henry Duncan was appointed Medical Officer of Health in Liverpool. Duncan combined private practice among the more affluent with the task of running dispensaries for the poor. It was in these dispensaries that he found all the results of poverty, squalor and inhuman living conditions that characterised the life in the cellars and the unhygienic courts where the marginal groups of Liverpool lived in the 1840s.

There seems to be little information about Duncan as a person, but the fact that among colleagues working in the dispensary, only Duncan seems to have been stirred to action on behalf of the poor, tells us something very important about him. The misery and the inequality was something he could not accept but had to do something about.

When, as we would interpret it, his conscience and his compassion were stirred he was stimulated to action. The action seems to have been planned and systematic as public health or community health action should be. It was dealing with what one might call the three classical 'Ps' in public health – the Public, the Politicians or decisions-makers and between them the Professionals.

Solidarity for Health

Similar processes led to the decision in 1977 among the world's public health leaders to embark on a Strategy of Health for All 2000. This was an expression in the health field of the general movement towards increased solidarity and sharing that grew out of the late 1960s and early 1970s. Even if the decision-making in the governing bodies of WHO seemed to be far away from the student barricades of 1968 and the green movements of the 1970s, it nevertheless drew its strength from the same source: the concern for solidarity, equity and human justice. This is the reason why the 'FOR ALL' is central to the process.

The gap between the haves and have-nots in health was considered unacceptable by the international leadership in health and a concerted action to do something about it was unanimously accepted. It was also accepted that Primary

Health Care (PHC) is the key to the achievement of this goal and the International Conference in Alma-Ata in 1978 was the focal point for these forces that basically were concerned with health and democracy.

The countries of Europe play different roles in this Health For All (HFA) and PHC process. Some brought their own experience of renewal and reform in public health and health care, others their plans and their dreams, while others came along because it seems to be the right thing to do (and perhaps because WHO resolutions did not seem to be so important in any case!) – but those European countries that were looking seriously at their own situation noted many differences and inequalities in the health status and health prospects of their people. Geographic as well as demographic risk groups were and are evident and some groups suffer from the summary effect of multiple risks, just as in Duncan's days.

Looking forward

What about the Year 2000 as a goal? The Cynics are making ironic remarks about WHO wanting to eliminate all illness by the Year 2000. Others suggest we adopt the Ethiopian calendar where in 1986 they have their year of 1979, and this would give us seven more years up to 2000!

Nobody had, of course, intended or dreamed that we could reach total absence of illness in 2000, but public health, action for the health of people, has always needed a forward-looking attitude, an attitude of hope, of improving things. Without hope there can be no public health. That is why today so many public health and community health people also are involved in activities to prevent nuclear holocaust, the ultimate public health problem of our day.

In many parts of Europe the prospective and forward-looking '2000' has stimulated people's imagination and inspired them to reflection, discussion, planning and action. Sometimes this has been, and is, in the form of 'scenarios'. What would we like the situation to look like in the year 2000 regarding traffic deaths/injuries, cancer, cardiovascular disease, infant mortality, suicides, etc? Many people, lay and professional, are involved in groups working on such 'mini-scenarios', that later are amalgamated to 'maxi-scenarios' as inputs to national HFA-strategies. There are examples of these at the local and area level here in Merseyside, in Bloomsbury in London, in Powys in Wales, in Denmark, Holland, etc. There are also national scenarios in several countries. The perspective of 2000 is working, wherever people care about health.

Disease and dis-ease

That health is more than the absence of disease has been a community health message for a long time. Health is also more important than disease and can only be understood and fruitfully promoted if we accept that disease usually is a symptom of 'DIS-EASE'. That disturbances and imbalances, social, economic and political lead to disease, was evident to Duncan, Chadwick, Simon, etc., and from them to those who wrote the Black report and many other reports influencing thinking and action for PHC and HFA. That is why we need a total view of health.

Realising that Duncan did not have a germ theory-oriented approach, one has claimed that he did the right thing for the wrong reasons – in improving housing, water supply and sanitation. It would be equally true to say that he had the right reasons to act against the obvious DIS-EASE that was at the root of the diseases that he saw but did not, could not understand (as we think we do). In today's 'WHO-slanguage' we might say that Duncan 'promoted overall health development through intersectoral action with emphasis on social, economic and political factors'. (With that he could have been used as a WHO consultant or member of an Expert Committee!).

Health for All in Europe

The process started rather slowly, almost reluctantly, but has then picked up speed in many ways. The first step was the development of a HFA strategy for Europe as a regional response to the global development. This strategy for Europe took a rather radical departure by establishing the following strategic approach. First, lifestyles conducive to health, i.e. what individuals are able to do, and should do, to preserve and promote their health. Secondly, as a collective responsibility to reduce or eliminate preventable hazards. Thirdly, availability of an appropriate service for care and cure. This area is, of course, very important but is preceded in the strategy by an emphasis on lifestyle and collectively preventable hazards. Different aspects of people's involvement run through all three areas. Intersectoral action is essential to deal with preventable hazards and the priority issues of cost containment and technology assessment are part and parcel of the system of care.

European Health for All Strategy

The European HFA Strategy also emphasises the prerequisites for health, employment, political stability, peace and better use of our common resources.

Primary health care as a key to HFA/2000 has, also in Europe, led to an analysis of the essential elements of PHC.

Education for health

Duncan was a pioneer for all public health communicators. He realised the importance of lay audiences (people with power) and lectured to the Literary and Philosophical Society where no doubt the decision-makers of his day came together. He also published his lectures as pamphlets for wider distribution and information.

All over Europe there is today a rapidly growing interest and emphasis on communication for health, health education, health promotion, health advocacy and heath literacy. My own definition is 'responsible sharing of information about health and disease'. The same information in different 'packages' for different audiences, the public, the politicians and the professionals.

Food and nutrition

National food and nutrition policies are developed, but the whole area is still full of uncertainties if not confusion. This aspect is unforgivably weak in the programmes of most medical schools and schools of public health. Public health officers/nurses or community health practitioners are losing out to other professions, and what is worse, to popular propagandists and charlatans who thrive when professional development lags behind or is confused.

Environmental health has today and tomorrow many more aspects than water and sanitation although these remain major areas of concern also in Europe. In major cities, public health people discuss whether the municipal tap water has been through three, six or nine kidneys.

Duncan, or Liverpool, did not know bacteria or viruses but he fought typhoid and cholera with environmental measures. He also was, like his colleagues, very much concerned with the 'miasma' – theory of their day. We tend to smile as we read about the miasma ideas, but we might as well ask ourselves: 'Where are our 'miasmas' in the 1980s? Which are our false preoccupations, basic misunderstandings and subsequent false priorities and mistaken action? Is it our idolatry of repair medicine or our unrealistic expectations regarding planning, health promotion and PHC?' There will be public health people in the future, analysing and critically judging both our action and our non-action in the latter part of the twentieth century.

Maternal and Child Health (MCH)

In many European countries, our findings attempt to change the content of the regular MCH contacts to concern for families with one parent, as well as two or more as a result of divorce, etc. adding new dimensions to traditional MCH activities.

Immunisation remains an important issue not only because of AIDS and other new diseases, but also the 'old' communicable diseases.

Prevention and control of endemic diseases in Europe focuses attention on cancer, cardiovascular disease etc.

Development of appropriate treatment for diseases and injuries

Manuals for specific diseases diagnose-related groups, monitoring and evaluation, technology assessment are among the issues currently receiving attention in Europe.

Provision of essential drugs

This is also of concern in Europe where several countries have developed lists of essential drugs and/or are steering the development through providing essential drugs free or through subsidised prices.

Primary Health Care and Health for All in different parts of Europe

First, some general principles. In general health development, two main areas can be distinguished. Firstly, the development of medical and health technology both for cure and care, prevention, promotion and rehabilitation. Public health professionals in Europe should be and are concerned about this development that may be compared to increasing the quality and quantity of the water in a water tank. Without appropriate technology, PHC-activities suffer and radical technological breakthroughs change, as we all know, the practice both of curative medicine and public health.

But it is also a major concern that existing technology is not being available to all those who need it or is used inappropriately resulting, among other things, in waste of valuable resources. The second area of using/applying technology is, therefore, receiving increasing emphasis in Europe. This may be compared to the pipelines, the network of water pipes and taps to carry the water from the tank.

We are emerging from a period of dependency, almost idolatry, of new medical technology and are beginning to assess more critically this technology. If for no other reason, this is done because the Finance Authorities are asking for such evaluation. They are demanding explanations about the use and results of resources provided to the health sector.

But together with these two main areas of concern we can also discern three major 'streams' of health development determining PHS and HFA in Europe. First, there is the age-old stream of individual medical care that has been so profoundly influenced by the technological developments in this century. This stream has aspects of medical technology interwoven with systems of training, remuneration, social security, social and health policy, administration and cultural traits that vary from nation to nation as well as within the same nation or country. In Europe, there is the whole spectrum from rigidly centralised medical care to heterogenous and pluralistic systems defying any form of 'systems management'. All this influences PHC and HFA processes.

The second stream might be called traditional public health with some roots going back a very long time but essentially stemming from the early part of the last century – from Duncan's days. Environmental health, food hygiene and the control of communicable diseases are here the well-known ingredients. Political, economic and social aspects have been involved but not in the same way as in the third stream, the new public health.

In some ways, the new public health is not really new but the old ingredients mixed and emphasised in new ways. This is both structural and regular, e.g. through local government, health councils, etc. and also less structured, more 'green' through patients' organisations, spontaneous pressure groups, etc.

The new public health is also more openly 'political' as health and human welfare are increasingly planned, steered and financed through public resources with the necessary mechanisms for decision-making. Health hazards and health goals are also more widely discussed and brought to the attention of political decision-makers.

The increasing public and political aspects create new situations for the public health professionals. This is no doubt one of the reasons why we find ourselves with new terminology, such as, community health, social medicine, health promotion, PHC, etc.

Differences within Europe

The three streams are each developed differently in different parts of Europe and their respective interaction is also different. Historical and political processes have their influence and so have social and cultural factors, including education. Different economic systems and models of financing are determining the health care models, the role of health workers, etc., that are really only a function of the general determinants stated above. Realising the risks of generalisation, I would, nevertheless, like to attempt an overview of recent public health development in Europe in terms of PHC and HFA.

Primary health care policies and practices are developed and attempts are made to meet the challenges for a new public health. Political changes have often been a necessary prerequisite for this new community or public health climate. The public health development in Southern Europe is well worthwhile following.

The developing countries of Europe are on the one hand certain areas of many European countries especially in Southern Europe, but I would also include Turkey, Morocco (and until 1984, Algeria) that are members of the European Regions of WHO. Within WHO, they bring into the European discussion and experience an important element of developing country challenge with poverty, ignorance, inequality of a kind the other countries may not really have seen since the days of Duncan.

The highly industrialised countries of western and continental Europe are pluralistic and many of them with federal structures that make it more difficult to develop or get acceptance for more systematic health policy and health development. Pluralistic systems of both providing and financing of care tend to support and emphasise medical care alone. Traditional public health efforts are, however, greatly helped by the general socio-economic development with positive effects on health. But this same development and its solutions also bring about the new problems that start crying out for 'new public health' processes.

In affluent industrial Europe, PHC and HFA meet on the one hand cynical critics and even primitive aggressive reactions in some medical journals. On the other hand, the general public, their organisations and the political leaders are more and more asking for new public health measures. This may be against radioactive contamination, toxic waste, polluted air, acid rain, or dying forests. Unfortunately, the medical profession, including some public health professionals, seem to be almost outsiders in this process. Where are the Duncans, the Simons and the Virchows today?

In Western Europe the United Kingdom is, as usual, in a special situation. On the one hand, the UK has its own public health history related to its role as social laboratory for industrialisation and subsequent public health development. On the other hand, it is (and especially Scotland, my friends there would say) a part of 'North Sea Europe', with the Netherlands and the Nordic countries. In these countries social policy, public health, and PHC developments have, to a large extent, a common historic and political tradition. Taking a risk in this company, I would like to throw out a question and a challenge with regard to the UK's role in public health. Are you going to continue your leadership role in public health or relinquish it across the North Sea or across the Atlantic?

Central Europe is an interesting entity with an identity, including a common public health tradition going back a long time. I am referring to the two Germany's, to Austria, Switzerland (partly), but also to Poland, Czechoslovakia, Hungary and Yugoslavia. For several hundred years, mainly through the German language, a common culture, science and higher education were developed including a shared medical and public health tradition. The Nazi-era of 1933–45 interrupted this traditional relationship which had its effects in the public health field, not only in the two German states but also in the other countries. The German public health tradition is only now being slowly rebuilt, coinciding with a new stirring of the old Central European identity.

This may be a necessary prerequisite to deal with the Central European severe environmental problems that refuse to respect the present boundaries between political entities or systems. The early signs of cooperation in battling common health hazards, such as air and water pollution, will have to overcome formidable political barriers but the challenge to develop a new public health will not go away and it remains to be seen how the constellation of public-politicians-professionals will meet this challenge in central Europe.

To differentiate in absolute terms between Central and Eastern Europe is, of course, not possible. Poland, USSR, Hungary and even Yugoslavia are partly in Eastern Europe and many people and institutions in the Soviet Union, Bulgaria and Rumania have traditionally shared some Central European links and heritage. The countries in Eastern Europe, not least due to the devastation during the 1939–45 war, extensively developed their medical care systems in the post-war period resulting in considerable improvement in the health status of their population. This, on the other hand, has led to over-dependence on a rigidly structured medical care system, that finds some difficulties in meeting new challenges. Traditional public health has also developed but, together with new public health measures, it has to compete with the economic priorities of industrialisation. This tension, common to all of Europe, has its special aspects in the centralistic socialist countries.

The Nordic countries, small in size and with a homogenous population, where social consensus can be reached more easily, have developed their mixed systems in a climate of relative social and economic stability.

A potentially dangerous over-dependence on medical care was compensated by the indirect positive health effects of rapid socio-economic improvements and increasing affluence. Today, the new public health is rapidly developing in all Nordic countries, and e.g. Sweden and Finland, presented national HFA Strategies to the respective Parliaments in 1985. They follow very much the European Strategy outlined above.

Health Challenges in Europe

Primary health care in Europe has, however, until now largely been understood as primary medical care. This again, in most European countries, is technically and financially heavily dependent on doctors. But there are also examples of shared responsibility with nurses and other non-medical professions and also signs of people's involvement, self-help and self-care. The systems of remuneration and social security often forms a serious obstacle to renewal either in attitudes or action.

The proliferation of citizens' groups, 'green' health movements for alternative care, etc., are signs of dissatisfaction with the existing systems. There are also signs of the need for a new public health in Europe, for which PHC and HFA are trying to be both symbols and examples.

One of the greatest and most difficult challenges in Europe is for intersectorial and interprofessional action. We have solved the problems that can be solved by one profession or within one sector of society. The problems, in whose midst we are and that are threatening our health and our future, are caused by multiple forces and need multiple, combined analysis and intervention. This is the challenge to public health in Europe.

In the industrial countries, the rising cost of health and especially medical care is demanding attention. Cost containment together with realistic technology assessment have, on the other hand, turned into an entry point for reflection and action regarding present and future health and health care systems. The resource question is forcing, also in pluralistic societies, hitherto reluctant partners to sit around the same table – searching for the new solutions.

When, in such discussions, primary health care for various reasons is less acceptable as a term, health promotion has proved to be an acceptable concept that is easily understood and can be given different content in different situations. Health promotion also seems to be more easily accepted for intersectorial collaboration where fears of medical domination and privileges often are a serious obstacle.

The European HFA Strategy is now expressed in the form of 38 targets, some for 1990, some for 1995, and others for 2000 (and beyond). The targets are grouped under the headings:

Adding years to life
Adding health to life
Adding life to years

A series of indicators have also been developed to monitor and evaluate the development in HFA and PHC in Europe.

Several countries have developed their national strategies and others are in the process of doing so. Health for All and PHC are a challenge to public health in Europe. A popular version of the European HFA Strategy is called 'Crisis 2000' and there are many signs that there will be a crisis if we do not succeed in developing a new public health strategy and praxis.

On the State of the Public Health*

Public Health (1988). 102, 431 437. E. D. Acheson, Chief Medical
Officer, Department of Health and Social Security. © The Society of
Community Medicine, 1988.

The title 'On the state of the public health', in addition to the obvious
meaning, happens also, for many years to have been the name of the
Annual Report of my predecessors and myself. From 1856 to the present day
these have formed an almost unbroken series of the Nation's health, its sickness
and mortality. Cholera and sanitary reform; smallpox and vaccination; slums;
malnutrition and infant mortality; venereal disease as it used to be called;
fluoridation; smoking and health; alcohol abuse; and most recently road accidents, skoal bandits and AIDS. All these and many more, some as success
stories; others downright failures; others as successes still to come; walk across
the pages.

In this spirit, I will first give my topic an historical perspective; and because
in my current post I seem to be squeezed in somewhere between Government,
the public and the medical profession, I will touch particularly upon the
contribution of central Government to good health. I will conclude with some
remarks upon health education and promotion.

There is another lecture which I might have given which I fear some of you
will have hoped to hear but will be disappointed. This would have tried to
evaluate the country's present state of health in comparison with its past health
and with the health of other countries. In these days when ill health depends
to such a large extent on personal behaviour – which in turn is influenced by
the economic and social environment and the political climate – the interpretation of such comparisons, however rigorous, would be extremely complex.

In any event I think all of us could hazard a guess at the conclusions. They
would be within the middle range of Headteacher's Reports:

> Has made creditable progress in some subjects but has certainly no good
> reason for complacency. Must concentrate more on the subjects he finds
> difficult.

It would be certain that we would conclude that much hard work was needed
on the following: Tobacco, alcohol, accidents, unhealthy diet, physical inactivity,
drug abuse and sexually transmitted disease. We would also probably conclude
that the old slums with their overcrowding, lack of ventilation and washing

---

* The fourth Duncan Lecture, delivered at the University of Liverpool, 11 February 1987

facilities, and unsafe water had been replaced by new slums in which the roots of ill health are more subtle and the outward signs of these include vandalism and graffiti.

I think of tobacco, solvent and drug abuse, coronary heart disease, lung and cervical cancer, and unwanted pregnancy as problems particularly prevalent in, but by no means exclusive to, these areas. We would also agree to the importance of some other new problems relating, for example, to the preservation of the health, independence and dignity of the very old. Here, unfortunately the ideal of a partnership of mutual support operates only too rarely as half of the very elderly live alone.

And of course we face a grave new problem in an old category; a new sexually transmitted disease, AIDS. I do not intend to expand on the problem of AIDS and of the virus HIV, which underlies it, but although we have so far in this country suffered slightly fewer than 700 cases there are good reasons why AIDS has already won an unchallengeable place among the major problems faced since the Reports on the State of the Public Health began in 1855. As did cholera in the nineteenth century, in an entirely different way, it will undoubtedly change the face of society. Although it is indeed a grave problem I am certainly not without hope. In developed countries like the UK at least, we have the means immediately to reduce greatly its rate of spread and in the longer term I have faith that human ingenuity, through science, will find a solution.

At this point I would like pay tribute to the powerful initiatives in respect of health promotion in this Region in which the Health Authorities and the University Department of Community Health cooperate. I venture to believe that William Henry Duncan would have approved of the twelve priorities for action in health promotion in the Regional Health Authority's strategic plan; and also of the travelling health fair with its fleet of buses. I was intrigued to hear that Duncan's favourite pub had been transformed into a 'public health theme pub' and wondered what activities take place there.

As far as the Government's role in health is concerned those of us who spend the first hour or so on Monday morning reading the weekend's newspaper cuttings on health topics soon recognise that, in the UK, expectations about the Government's contribution to good health are very considerable.

Among the most obvious of the expectations people have of the Government's contribution are the following:

(1) A competent GP (prepared to visit at home, if necessary).

(2) An emergency hospital service (rarely questioned).

(3) Timely elective treatment in hospital (not always timely).

(4) Care for the frail (physical and mental, young and old, at home or elsewhere).

But there are others, at least as important, which are often forgotten. Safe water and food; clean air, safety at work; control of infectious diseases; advice on how to stay well; early detection of treatable illness. Within the UK the central Government is expected to make a major contribution to all of these.

How has it come about that Government has bitten off quite as much? A

Government's first duty is often stated to be the protection of the State from attack by external enemies – and historically this doubtless was the prime function of the leader of the primitive tribe – and later the King's Government. But organised action by Government to protect society from at least 2 events with a major bearing on health did not come far behind. These were famine and pestilence which so often followed war and dissolution as depicted in Durer's famous engraving of the four horsemen of the Apocalypse. The Book of Exodus in the Bible mentions what effectively were State controlled granaries set up to prevent famine when, as sometimes happened, the annual inundation of the Nile failed. Perhaps this was the first contribution of a Government to good health.

The idea of isolation of persons suffering from infectious disease or quarantine arose when the first outbreaks of the Black Death were seen to result from the arrival of ships from the East. Legislation followed. Within the UK the history of the development of the Government's contribution to good health can be divided into 3 phases:

The first phase, up to 1919

This was the era when Government under the powerful stimulus of smallpox and cholera first took a grip on health policy. It included separate piped sewage and drinking water, the triumph of the microbial theory of disease and the beginning of effective vaccination and immunisation. Most of the successes were achieved by legislation enshrined in the early Public Health Acts. This led to the belief that most diseases might be due to the action of a single necessary agent, which if removed would lead to the control of the disease.

The second phase, 1919–1948

This phase opened with the setting of the Ministry of Health which brought together most Government functions in relation to health under one Minister answerable for health in the House of Commons. The Ministerial duties were defined as 'to take all such steps as may be desirable to secure the preparation, effective carrying out and co-ordination of measures conducive to the health of the people'. The optimism of that period of reconstruction immediately following the first World War springs from the text – 'All such steps as may be desirable' – not such steps as may be expedient or reasonable within the constraints. How enviable!

This was the period when, to public health by means of legislation and its enforcement, were added the improvement of health by the provision of personal services e.g. for mothers, babies and schoolchildren including of course immunisation. But there is more to come. As early as 1919, Central Government was issuing advice on health with far reaching implications on what it was necessary to eat to ensure optimal growth in children and good health in adult life. The classical work at Cambridge had identified the key role of vitamins and minerals. The advice emphasised, for the first time, that milk and green vegetables were rich in these essential nutrients and gave practical guidance about amounts – a pint of milk a day for the growing child – and about cooking, e.g. how cooking quickly destroys vitamin C.

In the 1930s surveys by Boyd Orr and Cory Mann demonstrated the link between poverty and malnutrition and the gross inadequacy of the diets of many British children. Further Government action followed, for example the provision of free school milk. But, ironically, it required the crisis of World War I to secure, through the food rationing system, a general and substantial improvement in the diet of children, and to ensure that rickets and scurvy became rare diseases. Information and education were insufficient. Policies were also needed. The period between the World Wars was the heyday of the Medical Officer of Health (MOH). Many of central Government's health policies were implemented through the medical departments of the local authorities and the School Medical Service with the MOH as the executive agent.

Although the Chief Medical Officer (CMO) had no management line with the MOH, in those days there were clear lines of communication and reserve inspectorial powers. The annual report which MOHs were required to publish were scrutinised carefully at the Ministry in Saville Row and were, I understand, occasionally followed up by what we would now call a 'site visit'. The Ministry also prescribed the main subject which should be covered in these reports. By the end of our second period, therefore, advice had been added to legislation and services as instruments of government policy for health. In fact some quite interesting health education campaigns had been carried out – for example – a campaign of posters, radio talks and local teach-ins emphasising the positive aspects of wartime food rationing. But there had also been another much more adventurous departure. In 1941, my predecessor Wilson Jameson broke new ground by being the first Civil Servant to give a Radio Broadcast. At peak listening time after the 9.00pm news he broached a topic which had previously never been discussed in the Press or Radio other than in heavily disguised terms, that of venereal disease, as it was then called. William Jameson had broken a taboo. There was favourable press comment and the whole question was opened up for discussion.

The third phase, 1948 to the present

The current era, from the perspective of Central Government, can properly be called the era of the National Health Service. The National Health Service dominates the work of the health side at the Department of Health and Social Security. Its sheer scale; its cost; its complexity; the public's expectations of it, but above all the fact that because it is 100% centrally funded, Ministers are directly accountable to Parliament for every penny, make sure of that. Although the hospital services as a cost per head of population have grown remarkably over the last 40 years, it is generally accepted that British health services are more cost effective than those in any other developed country. But the demands on it continue to grow. So we must continue to make every penny count. The present era is also sometimes properly referred to as the era of effective therapy. It is certainly an era when the advance of science and technology has multiplied the ways in which we can intervene to reduce the effects of illness and sometime to cure it. Antibiotics, psycholeptics, hypotensives to name but three have helped many. To those must now be added transplantation, joint replacement, lithotripsy, and the new diagnostic imaging techniques.

But as my main theme is the prevention of ill-health, not its treatment I will limit myself to one issue. High technology medicine is sometimes depicted as being in conflict with the promotion of health; and treatment as being in conflict with prevention. I do not see a conflict except in two aspects: where complex techniques waste money on ineffective procedures; and where treatment of a condition – cirrhosis of the liver or lung cancer – draws away attention from the eradication or control of the cause. And who can honestly say that both these do not sometimes occur? But many of the interventions which are available to us are highly effective. If not to save life, to make it more tolerable. Which one of us would not, if necessary, avail himself (or herself) of laser treatment to stave off diabetic blindness, a hip replacement, a coronary vein graft or a renal transplant?

So from the point of view of health, the present era, (and so far as we can see it, the future will be similar) is relatively speaking a scientifically well informed era where we have an increasing number of options. As many of these options are costly, we have to make choices and those choices must be better informed in respect of both outcome and cost; and the delivery of the service must be timely, efficient and sensitive. This in my opinion calls for a multi-disciplinary effort guided by medically informed management. At this point I leave diagnosis and treatment and return for the time remaining to the further-ance and promotion of health. As well as the era of the National Health Service and of effective treatment, our present era can be regarded as one in which the personal behaviour of individuals is the dominant factor in much ill-health; and also one in which many of the prevalent illnesses – cancer, coronary heart disease, stroke – are the results of not one 'necessary and sufficient cause' but many interacting factors.

My brother Roy, for whose work I often get the credit, has pointed out that illnesses against which the population can be protected without any element of behavioural change or choice are rare indeed.[1] The benefits of the Clean Air Act on chest disease is perhaps the last great piece of environmental legislation involving what he calls primary protection where injurious influences have been removed from our environment without any significant disturbance of our personal behaviour or effort on our part (except possibly the sacrifice of the pleasure of seeking a friendly coal fire in every grate). But how do we as a nation, and, in particular, how should the Government respond to the challenge that much of the incapacitating disease and premature death of the present time and the future can only be prevented by individuals making choices which alter their behaviour? I return to underline a point made earlier in which seven factors were listed, all of which involved personal choice, which together account for a large proportion of premature death and disability.

The best account I have seen of these issues comes from a speech by the Health Minister of Canada the Hon Jake Epp given at the Conference on Health Promotion in Ottawa last September.[2] This remarkable speech which was televised throughout Canada, and which is well worth reading, starts as I suspect many of us would in this room, from the standpoint of three challenges, namely that:

(1) Various forms of preventable disease undermine the health and quality of life of many people

(2) Many disabled people have insufficient community support to help them cope.

(3) Disadvantaged groups have poorer than average health.

To face these three challenges three strategies are proposed:

– fostering public participation

– strengthening community health services.

– co-ordinating 'healthy' public policy.

Strengthening community health services is such a topical subject in Britain and such an obvious need where chronic disability and the frail elderly present such major problems that I do not need to labour it. The idea of 'fostering public participation' about health is in a different category, however, because we have not yet really taken it on board as a policy issue. It incorporates but goes beyond education and health. Well produced, lively, accurate information about health like the popular 'Pregnancy Book' produced by the Health Education Council (HEC) is an essential element in equipping people to preserve and improve their health. But information does not go far without active commitment from the recipient. What is required is a greater recognition of personal responsibility for health and a more active personal participation by men, women and children than we have so far achieved in this country – although it is beginning to happen. Getting commitment means that those of us in the health care professions must involve others on equal terms. More discussion and less lecturing!

But self-care, mutual aid, and information are by themselves insufficient to create a climate for health. There needs also to be co-ordination to create a climate for health. There needs also to be co-ordination of public policies over a wide range – including taxation, housing, transport, agriculture all with health in mind. It is no use advocating recreational exercise if there are no playgrounds or parks; or fat reduction, if foods are not labelled.

As far as taxation as a tool for health is concerned the Chancellor takes the health issue into account when he considers the excise duty on tobacco and increases in taxation have proved an effective tool in curtailing the use of tobacco. But all CMOs in recent times have urged Governments of different political hues to do more in respect of both tobacco and alcohol.

Taken together the three Canadian strategies are encompassed in what WHO refers to as health promotion – the 'process of enabling people to increase control over and to improve their health'. Where have we got to with 'health promotion' in Britain? I will mention three facts. An agency within government; independent criticism and advocacy and health sensitive policies.

As you all know, the Secretary of State, with the urgent need for a continuing campaign on AIDS in mind, has decided to wind up the HEC and is replacing it as a Special Health Authority within the National Health Service. This will be the Government's agency for health education. One hopes it will strengthen the voice for the prevention of illness and promotion of health within the NHS. This remains weak in some areas. But there are other important functions to be discharged in relation to Local Authorities, Schools, and to the public at large. We are finding in the enquiry into the public health function which I am chairing that in this field all is not well with the links between the health authorities and the elected local authorities.

The Secretary of State has said that he expects the new Health Education Authority to exercise 'the same sort of sturdy independence' as the HEC. But at least one body with a fearless, totally independent voice outside Government should be available to pose the politically embarrassing question, or point to the awkward deficiency. Historically the Society of Medical Officers of Health in a corporate sense discharged this role. The weight of their authority was such that they forced important innovations on successive governments including the compulsory notification of infectious disease; and the provision of services for the control of tuberculosis. Today this function is split between the Royal College of Physicians, the other Colleges, Government funded bodies like ASH and Alcohol Concern, the BMA and the College of Health, all of whom do good work. Is this splintering inevitable? Should the Faculty of Community Medicine try to take up the mantle of the Society of Medical Officers of Health? Or have we reached a time when an exclusively medical organisation cannot fill the bill and as Richard Smith, Assistant Editor of the British Medical Journal has suggested we need a 'Public Health Alliance'.

Both in the Canadian Health Minister's speech and in WHO's Health for All Policy, stress is laid on the need for Government Departments other than those with the primary role in Health to make their contribution. In other words, and I quote 'all sectors of national and local government (should) take health considerations fully into account at the planning stage of new developments'.

In Whitehall there are already mechanisms at both Ministerial and official levels which ensure that co-ordination of advice is a reality and co-ordination of policy possible. At the level of advice, the CMO is the focus of a number of expert advisory committees whose members he is responsible for appointing and whose advice to Government should be independent and authoritative. In general the advisory mechanisms seem to work fairly well, but as far as policy is concerned can health always be the primary and overriding interest as seems to be suggested in some recent articles on health promotion and the 'new public health'? After all, poverty is an enemy of health and the wealth of a nation depends on commerce, industry and trade, and education; defence also has its place in the firmament. There are inevitable conflicts within Whitehall on health – not only with the tobacco interest but between alcohol and safe driving and the dairy industry and a reduction in animal fat. Reading between the lines in my predecessors' 'Reports on the State of the Public Health' there have always been vested interests although their nature and identity have changed over the years.

Conclusions

The time has come when I must try to draw together the threads of this somewhat rambling discourse. I will boil it down to three points.

My first point concerns the role of Central Government in health. Today this role is enormous, perhaps almost overwhelming. Looked at in the perspective of the century and a quarter covered by the Reports 'On the State of the Public Health' the move to the centre has accelerated since 1948 and now includes virtually all health services as well as a responsibility for the implementation of many of the policies which impinge on health. 1948 and 1974 saw substantial reductions in the role of the local elected authorities in this area. I do not, nor would it be appropriate for me to, comment critically on this. I simply note it.

My second point relates to engaging the consumers to a much greater degree – better described as ordinary men, women and children – in commitment and decisions about their health. This, simply because of the nature of the ills from which we suffer now and will suffer in the future, is inevitable, if our health is to improve. It needs amongst other things a change in the attitudes and skills of professional health workers – including doctors – although I see the continuing need for a properly informed and trained public health doctor in every district.

And what of the primacy of health? I was much attracted by an article by Katherine Whitehorn in the Observer of 12 October last, entitled 'Is this really health?'. Reviewing as we have tonight the passage of events from 'An era when the greatest threats were germs and epidemics to (one in which we have) the utter luxury of dying from stress, sex, steaks and smokes,' she concludes that the basis for health does indeed embrace the whole human condition, lifestyle; social setting; employment; parental behaviour; religion even. Yes, even religion; in recent weeks Ministers have had talks with all the national religious leaders.

Surely one does not have to be a political scientist to conclude that an idea of health as all embracing as this, will be given as much or little importance as individual people themselves wish it to have. And in determining this priority, voices outside Government are as important as forces within it. But looking across the span of years there can have been few sayings more pleasing to a Chief Medical Officer than Benjamin Disraeli's dictum in 1877:

> The health of the people is really the foundation upon which all their happiness and all their powers as a State depend.

References

1. Acheson, R.M. (1986). An ecological approach to preventive medicine. *Journal of the Royal Society of Medicine,* 79, 636–638.
2. Epp, J. (1986). Speech given to an international conference on health promotion. Ottawa, Ontario. November 17th.

Politics and the Public Health*

Public Health (1989), 103, 263–279. David Player. Director of Health Development and District Medical Officer. South Birmingham Health Authority, Oak Tree Lane, Selly Oak, Birmingham, B29 6JF. © The Society of Community Medicine, 1989.

I t has been said that those who do not learn from history will merely repeat the errors of the past – I intend to go no further back than the nineteenth century and the work of Duncan, the first Medical Officer of Health and his colleagues. It was then that the United Kingdom led the world in the implementation of public health measures. The main causes of mortality were the infectious diseases. These diseases were almost completely eliminated, not by therapeutic chemical intervention but by measures taken by local authorities under statutory powers which altered the living and working environment of the mass of the people. Thus as a result of improved housing, clean water and improved sanitation, local authorities achieved massive changes in the public health. They were also responsible for the development of community based preventive primary care services, such as ante-natal care, district nursing, health visiting and child welfare clinics.

Of course medicine played an important part and it is unfair as well as incorrect to dismiss the effects of advances in immunisation and vaccination and the introduction of chemotherapy. Nevertheless it is indisputable that environmental changes played the most important part in the success story of the nineteenth century.

Another critical factor in this period was the statutory requirement that local authorities should appoint a Medical Officer of Health. Although appointed by the local authorities, the Medical Officer of Health could not be sacked without the approval of the Secretary of State. Dr Duncan of Liverpool took up his post as the first Medical Officer of Health on 1 January 1847. The status he established for the role was described as 'a power in the commonwealth'. It could also have been described as a power for the commonwealth.

Further points from which we could learn were (1) that the Medical Officer of Health was required to publish an annual report each year on the state of the public health and (2) local government was a democratically elected authority and one should not forget that they ran municipal hospitals, often woefully underfunded, well before the introduction of the National Health Service in 1948.

---

* The 5th Duncan Lecture, delivered at the University of Liverpool, 2 December 1987

Before leaving the nineteenth century, we should recall that alongside aggressive individualism and rapid economic growth, there were astonishingly high levels of violence, and appalling living and working conditions. In contrast, as we have seen, there was always a strong strand of social action linked to local democracy. It is not true that the nice guys always come last.

What of the present? There have been enormous improvements in general health in the last 100 years. Sensitive indices of health such as Infant Mortality and Perinatal Mortality rates have plummeted, Maternal Mortality rates have reduced so much that there is an internal enquiry in most maternity hospitals now if a mother dies. Children are taller and better fed and life expectancy in all groups has increased very substantially except in the 15–24 year age group where there is a worrying trend due mainly to young people drinking and driving.

Overall the news is good, but if we look more closely there are many unattractive features of the present public health.

The killer diseases are no longer the infectious diseases, but diseases related to the social environment and behaviour. Bad housing is still a health hazard, as are poor traffic and transport policies. Although we have had magnificent success with the Clean Air Act, other environmental pollutions threaten health. Occupational health has improved. We now no longer have children and women working in the mines, but it is a sad fact that the National Health Service, the largest employer in Europe with a million workers has a grossly deficient occupational health service. There are looming dangers to the purity of our water supply, not least privatisation.

The behaviourally related diseases such as coronary heart disease (CHD), lung cancer and emphysema, cirrhosis of the liver and alcohol related accidents are now killing prematurely over 300,000 people a year. That is almost as many civilians and service people killed in the five years of World War II. At this rate 'Health for all by the year 2000' will be premature death for nearly four million British people. I would say we have a battle on our hands with casualty figures like that.

The behaviours I am talking about are: smoking, poor diet, over-consumption of alcohol and accidents. These are the anti-health forces, the health antagonists or enemies of the people.

Smoking

Let us take some good news first about smoking. In 20 years the proportion of the adult population smoking has decreased from two-thirds to one-third. This has been most marked in males in the age group 35–54 has decreased by almost 30%. This is a great victory for the public health. Males in the same social classes in the same age group have also shown a decrease of over 20% in CHD rates since smoking is a major risk factor in coronary heart disease. So we know what to do and we know how to do it.

The bad news about smoking is that girls and young women are now starting more than boys and young men. We can predict with confidence that lung cancer will become the commonest cancer in women by 1990, displacing breast cancer at the top of this gruesome league. Part of the reason for this is the cynical, ruthless manipulation of the media through advertising and sponsorship by the tobacco industry. The messages beamed at women in the glossy magazines – three or four full page, full colour cigarette advertisements, the production of cigarettes aimed specifically at the female market – such as Virginia Slims and Kim sponsorship of sporting events aimed at women. Take the recent tennis tournament at Eastbourne shown on peak BBC TV sponsored by Pilkington Glass and by Virginia Slims. Both the winner, Sukhova, and the runner-up, Navratilova, when receiving their cups on BBC TV only mentioned the sponsorship by Virginia Slims. You know we must really see an end to this exploitation of our young people by those selling such deadly weapons. The tobacco industry will go to almost any ends to defend their so-called right to promote their product as witness what happened to Sir George Young, ex-Junior Minister of Health, and Joseph Califano, ex-Secretary of State for Health in the Carter administration. When I met the Tobacco Worker's Union some years ago, I sympathised with their lot but they would not even admit that cigarettes were harmful to health. 'There was no evidence' they said. Anyway, their industry was amongst the biggest export earners for this country and regularly received the Queen's Award to Industry. What this means is that Britain is now a net exporter of disease to the third world. Instead of importing cholera, typhoid and smallpox 100 years ago, we now export rapidly rising death rates from lung cancer and coronary heart disease.

Diet

We eat more than in the nineteenth century, but we are eating too much of the wrong things, namely, too much fat, too much sugar, too much salt, and not enough fibre. Wrong diet as another major factor in CHD has, however, been changing for the better in the last 4–5 years. This must be attributed to better health education, coincidental with the publication of the NACNE and COMA Reports. Following on, parts of the food industry have seen the light, not altruistically (heaven forbid) but because of the profit potential. There has been a revolution in supermarket shopping with an impressive choice now of low fat products, sugar and additive free products and an increase in high fibre products.

A good example is the deal the Health Education Council made with the Federation of Bakers. Three years ago the Health Education Council agreed to put its logo on all wrapped bread with the message that bread is high in fibre and is good for you, especially wholemeal bread. In return the bakers cut the salt content of all their bread by 12.5%. So, at a stroke, there was a significant decrease in national salt consumption. As far as sales of bread were concerned, the decrease which has been going on since the end of World War II stopped and sales are now rising. Importantly the sales of brown and wholemeal bread went up from 6% of total sales to 25%. A case of enlightened self-interest which improves the public health.

Alcohol

Alcohol abuse (important – not against alcohol *per se*) is more socially disruptive than anything else in our society as well as causing an estimated 20,000 deaths each year. In many of our leading hospitals 25% of acute admissions are related to alcohol abuse. Consumption has doubled within the past 30 years and associated harm has increased relatively. It is the main 'drug of solace' in our culture yet as an 'anti-health' force it is responsible for much cirrhosis, gastritis, malnutrition, psychiatric illness as well as being associated with road traffic accidents, domestic and workplace accidents, poor work performances, absenteeism, violent crime (50% murderers are under influence of alcohol, 50% of victims also) suicide, child abuse and divorce.

The alcohol industry spends over £100 million per annum on advertising and sponsorship of one kind or another. It is quite irresponsible in aiming some of this at young people; as the alcohol industry are doing at present using the shirts of soccer teams.

Like the nicotine in cigarettes, alcohol is an addictive drug, but this is seldom acknowledged. Indeed other addictive substances like heroin are treated quite differently by governments and professions. Last year the Government spent over £400 million combating heroin abuse including £17 million for advertising. There were less than 300 deaths. In the same year they spent (or allowed to be spent) approximately £1 million combating alcohol abuse of which £400,000 was spent on advertising. Why?

The industry is very powerful: it had more than 30 MPs in last Parliament who were paid consultants or benefited financially from association. The Chancellor collects about £5 billion in taxes from the alcohol industry. It is a very big employer of labour and it is a very profitable investment.

Alcohol abuse is much harder to combat than tobacco because nearly everyone drinks, don't they? The alcohol industry has also been brilliant in developing the myth that indeed a little alcohol is positively good for your health. I have reviewed the scientific evidence. It does not support this myth.

There have been attempts by the alcohol industry to set up joint schemes with health promoters to combat alcohol abuse. Well intentioned I am sure, but they have always broken down when the industry realises that our objective is the reduction in total and *per capita* consumption which is directly related to degree of harm, and their objective is an increase in consumption and increase in profit.

I have identified several 'health-antagonists' or 'enemies of the Public health' or 'Enemies of the People'. There are others and we must be aware of them, such as parts of the agricultural industry, of the pharmaceutical industry, of the nuclear power industry. Of particular concern is the disgraceful pay of the majority of the workers in the National Health Service. This is the time bomb

which could destroy our admired National Health Service. The numbers of
low-paid workers on Family Income Supplement is disgraceful.

Fairly recently there have been changes in local government and in the
national Health Service which have militated against the best interests of the
public health. 1974 saw the last of the Medical Officers of Health and the return
of most physicians concerned with community medicine behind the barricades
of the hospital walls. The National Health Service became increasingly concerned with treatment, care and high tech medicine. Not that this was bad in
itself – indeed there are many leading better quality lives as a result. But the
big killers have now been identified. We continue to pull people out too far
downstream without walking upstream to find out who or what is pushing them
in. As Professor Thomas McKeown said: 'The disposal of society's investment
in health is based on quite different premises. It is assumed that we are ill and
made well, whereas it is nearer to the truth that we are well and made ill.'

With local authorities in 1974 losing a part of their public health function,
although retaining Environmental Health, Social Work, Education, Recreation
and Leisure and Housing, there was a period of lessening interest in many
Town Halls in health in its broadest sense. However, since 1981 several large
local authorities, such as Sheffield, Greenwich, Oxford, Lambeth, Slough,
Nottingham, Leeds, Manchester and Birmingham have introduced health promoting initiatives and have formed Health Committees again (as distinct from
Environmental Health Committees) and appointed full-time Officers with a
health function, sometimes in association with the Local District Health Authorities.

This sort of thing is now widespread and progressing all the time. There has,
in fact, been a considerable rethinking of Public Health by many local authorities
already and a dynamism is very apparent. Like-minded local authorities meet
regularly and the Association of Metropolitan Authorities has created a new
health forum within its structure. Local authorities have also played a big part
in the genesis of the new Public Health Alliance, about which, more later.

In this section, looking at the present, I must dwell on two matters which
concern me. Firstly the tendency for many, including those in Government, to
blame the victims for their health related behaviour and to deny the importance
of the environment even on these 'personal behaviours' like smoking, abusing
alcohol and eating the wrong diet. This is not only morally and philosophically
unsound, it is a rationalisation of facts which they would rather not hear about
because they then might have to do something about it. It's related to the 'I'm
all right Jack' attitude. What this attitude allows is a de-politicising of public
health issues which is in keeping with the essentially anti-democratic nature of
the NHS.

The second matter I wish to emphasise is the growing divide in the country
between the rich and the poor. We are in 1987 a deeply divided nation. In the
last seven years the rich have become richer financially and the poor have
become poorer. (One fact – the number of children living in poverty has doubled
during this time). In health terms the 'Health Divide; Inequalities in the 1980s'

by Margaret Whitehead.[1] showed conclusively what many of us had feared. Since the Black Report of 1980, health inequalities between rich and poor had increased. For all causes of death, except perhaps skin cancer and breast cancer, the rates were higher in Social Class IV and V than in Social Classes I and II. Overall the health of the people has been improving but the gap between the have's and the have not's is wider. This is intolerable and I can only repeat my preface to the 'Health Divide':

> This final report from the Health Education Council before its demise on 31 March 1987 is, in my opinion, an essential element in the public debate which must occur on health inequalities in the United Kingdom.
>
> Such inequity is inexcusable in a democratic society which prides itself on being humane. To eliminate or even reduce it substantially would be a major contribution to the health of the people of this country.

We know that poverty is harmful to health and is the root cause of other factors which we include in terms like multiple deprivation, like poor housing, bad general environment, bad diets, poor heating. Before discriminating for those who already have, by such means as privatisation of industry, lower mortgage rates etc and privatisation of our health, educational and housing services, we must positively discriminate towards the poor and areas of multiple deprivation.

But I must spend more time on the 'Health Divide – Inequalities in Health in the 1980s'.

The Health Divide

Background

In 1977, the Labour Government commissioned a Research Working Group, chaired by Sir Douglas Black, to study inequalities in health and the policy implication of this. This Black Report,[2,3] which gave a picture mainly of the early 1970s, highlighted a serious situation and put forward 37 recommendations for action.

That stimulated a great amount of research and initiatives to deal with inequalities all over the country, so, in January 1986, as Director General of the Health Education Council, I commissioned Margaret Whitehead to update the Black Report to get a clear picture of what was happening in the 1980s. The intention was to publish this along with an update of the Court Report of 1976 on child health services (published in July 1987 under the title 'Investing in the Future') and with an update of the 1976 report 'Prevention and Health: Everybody's Business' (still awaiting publication).

Margaret Whitehead was given a deceptively simple brief: to update the evidence on inequalities in health and to comment on the progress made on implementing the recommendations in the Black Report. It was decided to follow the format of the Black Report closely, covering the same topics and issues with the most up-to-date evidence available. The aim was to bring together into one volume the findings of numerous research groups around the country, so as to act as a resource for a wide range of people, to aid their policy-making and day-to-day work. It was to include a comprehensive picture of inequalities in the 1980s, explanations of some of the research studies and techniques used, and plenty of references for those who wanted to follow up specific topics in greater depth.

The review was published by the Health Education Council in March 1987, with the title *The Health Divide: Inequalities in Health in the 1980s*. By 'inequality in health' we meant not just natural variation, but unfair or unacceptable inequality which could be considered preventable. This was in line with the comments of a World Health Organisation meeting in 1985. 'In health terms, ideally everyone should have the same opportunity to attain the highest level of health and, more pragmatically, none should be unduly disadvantaged!' [4]

Findings of 'The Health Divide'

(1) *The present pattern.* Serious and persisting social inequalities in health were found on many fronts. The picture emerges of those at the bottom of the social scale, however measured, having much poorer health and survival chances.

(a) Using occupational class as an indicator of social position, then the poorer health of the socially disadvantaged shows up not only in mortality statistics, but also in morbidity figures and most recently in indicators of positive health and well-being. It is apparent for most causes of death and also for the major diseases which are chronic and painful, but not life threatening like arthritis. Such inequalities in health are not limited to one period in life, but are evident from infancy to old age.

(b) There are some problems with using occupational class, but if the results are checked against other measures like housing tenure or car ownership, a consistent pattern of inequality is still seen. If we take housing tenure as an indicator of command of resources, financial security, credit-worthiness etc., owner-occupiers were seen to have lower mortality than private tenants, who in turn have lower mortality figures than local authority tenants. When lack of car is taken as a proxy for poverty, higher mortality is revealed in groups who do not have a car, with lower mortality for those with one car, and even lower mortality for those with two.

(c) *Unemployment and health.* Unemployment can be taken as yet another measure of social (and material) disadvantage. There have been more studies of a longitudinal nature since the Black Working Group reported, following the fate of individuals over a period of years as their employment circumstances change. Differences have been found in physical and mental health between the unemployed and those in work, for example, for men mortality is 36% higher in the unemployed than the average for all men. Their wives have 20% higher mortality. Attempted suicide rates are far higher in the unemployed compared to the employed – of the order 11:1 for men, and the risk increases with increasing length of unemployment,[5] see Table 1 below.

Table 1

Length of unemployment	Ratio of risk attempted suicide unemployed:employed
Less than six months	6:1
Six-twelve months	10:1
Over twelve months	19:1

Studies on mental health have documented the decline into depression and the increase in psychiatric illness as unemployment deepens, and the effect it can have not only on themselves but on their wives and children.

(d) *Regional differences.* The Black Report documented a clear pattern of higher mortality in the North and West of the Country and lower mortality in the South and East in the 1970s. This North South divide is still just as evident in the 1980s. For example, death rates among both men and women of working age are close to twice as high on Clydeside as in East Anglia.

A recent national survey (the Health and Lifestyle Survey) has now also provided information on various forms of illness and on health behaviour in the different regions. The pattern of illness was very similar to that for deaths, with higher rates in the North and North West for a whole range of diseases and restricting conditions, some of which would not figure highly in the death statistics but would be the cause of much misery and pain.

So it is true that there appears to be a clear North/South divide in health. But what is its significance? In the past six or seven years many studies have been carried out to look at the health profiles of much smaller areas than those Regions or Health Authorities. These small area studies reveal a much more complex picture. They find that communities living side-by-side in the same region can have widely different health profiles, with pockets of very poor health alongside pockets of much better health.

This led Greater Glasgow Health Board to report in 1984:

In several communities (in Glasgow) death rates were as low (or lower) than in the healthiest countries in the world whereas in many others death rates are among the highest anywhere.

These pockets of poor health corresponded to areas of poverty and material deprivation, while the pockets of better health corresponded to more affluent areas. In the Northern Regional Health Authority, 65% of the difference in health between wards could be 'explained' statistically by deprivation indicators.

(e) *Ethnic minorities on health.* On this issue it has to be stressed that the official statistics are still inadequate for studying the health of ethnic minorities.

However, the available evidence does show some cause for concern. The death rates of babies in some ethnic groups are much higher than for the UK population as a whole, especially for babies born to mothers from Pakistan and Bangladesh. There are also high death rates in adults for some diseases, for example, CHD in immigrants from the Indian Sub-Continent, but also low rates for common diseases in the UK like lung cancer and bronchitis. High mortality from accidents in all immigrant groups is also causing concern. We really need to follow the health profiles through into the second and third generations but as yet this has not been done on a national scale.

(f) *Gender differences*. There is still the familiar pattern of women having lower mortality but higher morbidity than men. But if you start to delve deeper into the connections between employment, marital status, presence or absence of children etc., and health, then a far more complex picture emerges, e.g., some groups of women living in disadvantaged circumstances suffer even worse health than men living in similar circumstances.

(2) *Trends*. The health of the population as a whole has continued to improve over the past decade – if measured in death rates, life expectancy, height, dental health etc. In fact mortality has been declining all this century.

But the point here is – have these improvements been experienced equally across all sections of the community or have some benefited more than others? Are some lagging behind? Is the health gap getting wider, narrower, or is it about the same? There are many technical problems in answering these questions. The Black Report reviewed evidence from 1931–1971 and concluded that the gap in health between the advantaged and disadvantaged had in some cases stayed the same, while in others it had become wider. What has happened in the decade from 1971? Certainly in adults of working age non-manual groups experienced a faster decline in death rates than manual groups, so the health gap widened. In some of the major killers, death rates increased for the manual classes while showing a decline in non-manual classes: for example, in coronary heart disease, the major killer in men, there was a 1% increase in mortality in manual men and a 15% decrease for non-manual men. In women, lung cancer and CHD mortality increased in manual classes, while decreasing in non-manual classes. In babies at birth and in the first month of life the health gap stayed the same, but for post-neonatal mortality the health gap decreased – a very welcome trend.

Trends in morbidity from 1974 show an increase in rates of reported illness (unlike death rates which are declining). Illness rates in manual groups have consistently been higher than in non-manual groups over the period from 1974–1984, and the gap between the two has increased over that time, particularly in the over 65 age group.

Similar trends are found using other indicators: from 1971–1981, there was a decline in mortality for degree-holders while no decline for those with no educational qualifications.

There are many problems with tracing longer-term health trends but recently there have been three re-analyses of the data from 1921–1971, which basically concluded that all classes have profited from the decline in mortality but higher status groups have profited more than most.

(3) *Use of health services.* What of equality in health care? Are we providing health services which are equally accessible and of equal quality for all social groups? The NHS was based on this principle. The Black Report suggested that access was in some cases biased in favour of non-manual socio-economic groups. What is the picture in the 1980s?

It is very difficult to get a comprehensive overview of what is going on. The evidence is very patchy. Since 1980 some studies have found no evidence of bias in favour of particular social groups in GP consultations, while others have found problems in physical access, differences in quality of care, less preventive use of the service by lower social groups and differences in the nature of illnesses presented to GPs and therefore in the requirements for treatment.

There is no doubt that disadvantaged groups use treatment services more than advantaged groups. What is not clear is whether their increased use matches their increased need or falls short of it. For example, in one General Practice, patients from a deprived area were matched with patients from an affluent area and compared.[6] Deprived patients had 60% more hospital admissions, 75% more casualty attendances, and almost three times as much mental illness, as the affluent group. The same trend was seen for physical illness, referrals and consultations, but there was more non-attendance for preventative care in the deprived group. In total, there was a 50% higher morbidity load to health services from the deprived group than from the affluent group. This reinforces the point that patients from deprived areas are in a high risk, priority category by any standards.

(4) *Explanations of inequalities in health.* The possible explanation for these continuing inequalities in health fall under four main headings:

(a) Artefact.

(b) Healthselection.

(c) Behaviouralculturalexplanations.

(d) Materialiststructuralistexplanations.

(a) *Artefact.* This suggests that what we are seeing in the statistic is not real. It is an artefact of the way mortality rates are calculated, of changes in the Registrar General's social class classification and of changes in the proportion of the population in each class. All these points have been examined recently and the social class gradient in health is still evident when they are all taken into consideration. The trends remain if particular occupations are followed over time, or if measures are used to take account of the changing size of classes. Social position can be measured by other methods and still the gap between the health of the favoured and the disadvantaged is seen. We can be confident that we are dealing with a genuine and serious problem.

(b) *Health selection.* This explanation suggests that the healthy move up the social ladder and the unhealthy move down – under this system the health gap is virtually inevitable and would persist indefinitely.

There is evidence that some health selection does occur. Those who are sick or disabled do have poorer employment prospects and are at greater risk of poverty than those who are well. One longitudinal study found that boys who were seriously ill in childhood tended to end up in a lower social class than would be expected from their family circumstances.[7] Taking height as a measure of health before marriage, it was found that taller women tend to be upwardly mobile at marriage and produce babies with a higher chance of survival.[8]

However, attempts to quantify the size of the health selection effect suggest that it only makes a small contribution to the overall health gap – i.e., it is not a sufficient explanation for the large differentials observed.[9]

(c) *Behavioural/cultural explanations.* This explanation accepts that social factors can affect health, but emphasises the difference in personal health habits and the life-style of individuals. The idea that people 'inflict' illness on themselves by smoking, drinking and poor diet is reinforced here. The fact that the poorer sections of society indulge in more damaging behaviour than the rich would explain the health gap in this case.

The evidence does indeed show that disadvantaged groups have an unhealthier life-style than the more advantaged members of society in such areas as smoking, heavy drinking, leisure-time activity and food. In 1984, for example, 17% of professional men and 15% of their wives smoked, compared to 49% of unskilled manual workers and 36% of women in this category.[10]

However, these life-style differences, while explaining some, cannot wholly account for all the observed inequalities because:

(i) inequalities are observed for diseases *not* related to smoking or any known risk factor,

(ii) inequalities in health are found between non-smoking groups, and

(iii) studies which control for behaviour still find excess mortality in the poorer groups. The British Regional Heart Study found that when smoking and drinking is controlled the risk of CHD is still much higher for unemployed men than for employed men.[11] In the Whitehall Study of civil servants,[12] there was a three-fold difference in CHD risk between the top and the bottom grades, which was reduced by less than one-third when the classic CHD risk factors were controlled. In the USA the Alameda County Study compared the survival chances of different income groups over eighteen years and again found that most of the excess risk of death in the poorer groups remained when 13 risk factors were taken into consideration.[13] Such studies show that the simple behavioural explanation is inadequate on its own, though it does play a part.

In recent years several studies have gone out into the community to test this assumption: to explore why people act in the way they do. Why do they eat lots of carbohydrates and fatty foods, for example, and why do they not bring their children for preventative care? In many cases such studies find that it is not ignorance or laziness which stands in the way of adopting a healthier life-style, but quite practical, down-to-earth obstacles, which would fit in with the following 'materialist' explanation.

(d) *Materialist structuralist explanations.* This explanation emphasises the role of differences in living and working conditions and their effect on health, as well as the importance of the structure of society and how it is organised. In support for this explanation there are strong correlations between ill-health and various indicators of social and material deprivation, housing and working conditions, and unemployment which remain when other factors are taken into consideration. The casual link between unemployment and deteriorating mental health has been shown in longitudinal studies following people as they move in out of employment. Studies of how income affects health have mainly been confined to indirect studies – which look at the influence of income on food choices and health behaviour as indicated in the previous explanation. Sometimes, for example, it is found that people take unhealthy action not out of choice, but out of necessity. Food is often used as a flexible item in the budget (unlike rent and rates) and food is cut down when money is short. Whether to take a child for a health appointment can hinge on transport time and financial considerations. Such studies really show the link between the behavioural and the materialist explanations. They provide fresh insight into the way behaviours are influenced by living and working conditions and argue for a policy which recognises the link between the two in preference to policies which focus solely on the individual.

The conclusion from the most recent evidence is still in line with that of the Black Report in 1980: socio-economic factors (including life-styles) play the major part in maintaining inequalities in health.

Responding to inequalities in health

The Black Report made 37 recommendations for policies to reduce inequalities in health covering research, health and social services, and local and national government. Note that, as the major source of inequalities was seen as material living and working conditions, the policy was not confined to the NHS but involved a wider strategy of improvements in many fields. It is important not to blame all inequalities on the failure of the NHS: it cannot be expected to solve the problem single-handedly. The 37 recommendations came under three main headings:

(1) *Research and information*

Improvements in collection of information on social factors and health.

(2) *Health and social service*

Priority for children.

Priority for disabled and elderly.

Priority for preventative and educational action.

(3) *The wider strategy*

Attack on child poverty.

Improvements in housing and working conditions.

Co-ordinated local and national government policy on health.

The response to these recommendations has been characterised by a lack of action at national level, with no commitment or lead taken to reduce inequalities by the Government, but by enthusiastic, if uncoordinated, action at the grass-roots level. *The Health Divide* documents the lack of progress, and in some cases, the decline in services that the Black Working Group wished to see built up, but in this paper the positive aspects are picked up – the initiatives which have been taken by individuals and organisations around the country to try to tackle the problem.

What has been done?

Initiatives come under eight main headings and examples of each type are given below:

(1) *Local monitoring of social factors and their effects on health*

'Local Black Reports' have been carried out by the Northern Regional Health Authority; by District Health Authorities in Grimsby, Sheffield,[14] Coventry, Bloomsbury, South Derbyshire, as well as Greater Glasgow Health Board[15] and Northern Ireland plus joint ones or local authority ones in Manchester, Sheffield, Merseyside and Bristol.

(2) *Relaying information to staff and training*

Greater Glasgow Health Board has produced an unemployment and health study pack which has been used for training purposes. The Health Education Council funded a project on the training needs of health visitors, health education officers and social workers in relation to unemployment and health. Another on the issues of health and race has been funded with the National Extension College and the DHSS.

(3) *Adapting services to suit those most in need*

Great progress has been made here to take account of transport difficulties. The Isle of Wight, Hounslow and Edinburgh have decentralised antenatal clinics. Some have mobile clinics: Southwark makes use of these to improve immunisation rates and Sheffield to improve cervical cancer screening in the most deprived areas. Ormskirk District takes child health services to outlying areas. Others use mini–vans to bring parents and children to central clinics. Bury Community Health Council (CHC) commissioned a study of the illness problems in one deprived estate and what the community really needed in the way of health care. The timing of clinics and the attractiveness of waiting areas have also been improved. In response to ethnic minority needs some districts like Tower Hamlets have been employing interpreters in antenatal and child care. Many also provide special diets in hospitals.

Some practice opportunistic health care. Bolton CHC and District Health

Authority (DHA) set up a pregnancy walk-in clinic in the centre of town staffed by a midwife. The Trades Union Congress and Spastics Society have pioneered work-place antenatal care projects in Scotland and Oldham. In Nottingham they have been experimenting with the reorganisation of child health clinics: extra health visiting has been provided for infants at risk of post-neonatal mortality because of their deprived living conditions. A general practice in the North East of England has been researching ways of reaching deprived patients with missed preventative care, taking every opportunity they can to offer preventive services.

(4) *Exploring the community development approach*

This approach aims to help deprived communities identify and act on their own health needs. Paddington and North Kensington Health Authority has funded a research project to examine the use of this approach in health visitors' work. The Greater Glasgow Health Board has funded several projects of this nature and one in Catford has looked at the feasibility of a CHC employing a health worker to help local people identify their health priorities.

(5) *Promoting the uptake of welfare benefits as part of an anti-poverty policy*

Somerset DHA has been training staff in welfare benefits. Manchester City Council has 20 'Health rights workers' advising on such issues and in Glasgow the current campaign to encourage uptake of benefits has led to a huge increase in claims. Some individual GPs (like Jarman in London) have recognised that advice on welfare benefits is a legitimate part of caring for their patients.

(6) *Building up community care services*

This is especially important so that elderly and disabled people can remain in their own homes. Cheshire Social Services Department has transformed its home-help service into a home-care service. The home-care assistants have extended roles along the lines envisaged by Black, carrying out simply nursing and social duties. Some health authorities and local authorities are getting together to rethink their policy for the elderly: in Hillingdon they have assessed the needs of all the elderly in the area and are now combining and expanding home-care and auxiliary nursing services, promoting neighbourhood and voluntary care, and accommodating in residential homes those people who really need it.

(7) *Providing a healthier environment*

Local authorities are really waking up to their health promotion potential. A survey in 1985 found that one-third of AMA members had some form of health committee, and the number is growing all the time. Manchester City Council called a consultation on the Black Report when it was first published and came up with a ten-point plan for immediate action including improving take-up of benefits, improving statistics on health at ward level, improving housing by tackling damp, plus smoking and nutrition policies. The council now has a 'Health Campaign Worker' to co-ordinate the activities with various agencies and a CMS focusing on housing and health inequalities, including access to services, pollution and community safety. Sheffield City Council has also been very active: it commissioned one of the most detailed 'Local Black Reports', has a food and smoking policy, and is developing a response to the WHO Healthy Cities project. Oxford City Council is perhaps the most active of all. It adopted a 'City Health Strategy' in 1986 – with the aim of reducing inequalities in many areas, such as in the housing department. Each council department has to produce health targets to focus their work on the overall goals of the health strategy and one hundred targets have so far been identified. The Planning Department is producing health profiles, there are also community development health projects in deprived areas of the city, and safe-cycle routes and community fitness programmes are being developed. As a major employer, the City Council is also developing a model occupational health policy. In short, many local authorities now recognise that they have a major contribution to make, even though they cannot solve the poverty problem themselves.

(8) *Raising awareness*

Many professional and voluntary bodies have been playing an important part by organising conferences and seminars to discuss what to do about inequalities in health. Some have been issuing discussion documents and 'charters for action' from their own particular perspectives, e.g. The British Medical Association, Faculty of Community Medicine and Health Visitors Association have all considered the subject seriously. The latest initiative in this field is the Public Health Alliance, launched in July 1987 to try to ensure that health is put on the agenda of all major policy discussions. Activity at the grass-roots is most encouraging. What we now want is a serious national commitment to Healthy Public Policy.

The future

It is now evident in the United Kingdom, as in other developed countries, that further investments in conventional medical care of acute and chronic illness will produce decreasing returns on investment. Ironically, the very success of the first public health revolution and medical advances have produced outcomes such as increased longevity which, increasingly, places an increasing burden on the carers (particularly of the very old in the community).

It is becoming increasingly obvious to professionals and politicians alike, that the second revolution in public health, or the new public health movement, must address itself, like the first revolution, to matters of the social environment and life-styles.

We, in this country, are not the first to make this conceptual breakthrough. Our colleagues in USA and Canada, in particular, following important reports by the Surgeon-General in the USA[16] and especially the Lalonde Report in Canada,[17] have made considerable moves towards a concept of health promotion, as distinct from health education. In my opinion, health education by itself is seldom effective. It needs to be combined with legal, fiscal, political and environmental action. The sum of all these parts I call '*Health Promotion*' or, as John Ashton would say, 'health promotion is anything you need to do to improve the health of people'.

Interestingly and relevantly, there followed substantially increased activity in the American Public Health Association and the Canadian Public Health Association. In 1985 the Kings Fund and Health Education Council sponsored a group of young health promoters on a visit to the United States of America and Canada. A report of this was published this year; edited by Christopher Robbins it is entitled 'Health Promotion in North America! Implications for the United Kingdom'. Significantly one of the main recommendations to emerge was the formation of a United Kingdom Public Health Association or Public Health Alliance.

The WHO has also been active in this debate and has nailed its colours to the mast by advocating four principles to improve the public health:

(1) Primary health care must be multisectoral.

(2) There should be sparing, judicious use of high tech medicine.

(3) There should be community participation (and that includes determining the perceived needs of the community).

(4) Equity.

WHO has also set all countries the task of Health For All by the Year 2000 and, importantly, set a list of 36 targets. The United Kingdom Government is a signatory to this.

What then of the future for public health in the United Kingdom? Firstly, what should not be done. Let's have no victim blaming. The ideal of public health requires public commitment to health rather than a shift of responsibility to the individual. Efforts to place all the responsibility on the individual detracts attention from the role of national government and local government in promoting the public health. No account is taken of how each individual makes the decisions, which determines the quality of his or her life-style. An underfinanced trickle of blandishments about smoking, drinking or nutritional behaviour can have little impact when received against a tidal wave of advertising and promotion by those associated vested interests which, in Peter Draper's words, 'poison our thinking water'.

Many pre-election opinion polls at the last General Election reflected great public concern about health, indeed health was the number one topic. Yes, the DHSS remains a low-status Government Department – clearly a paradox between the public and Government perception about the importance of health. The recent establishment of a Cabinet Sub-Committee on AIDS is of great public and historical moment. It's the first time this century that a public health topic has assumed such importance and has shown real Government commitment to public health. During my time as Director-General of the Health Education Council, the Council was asked to submit evidence to the Acheson Enquiry on the future of Community Medicine. One of our recommendations was that the importance of health should be recognised and that it should be considered by a Cabinet Sub-Committee, reflecting the role each Government

Department has in the promotion of health. Truly the main decisions about health will be taken at the Cabinet table, not the operating table.

What else should we be doing?

We need then an independent source of advice on the public health. Local authorities have an enormous part to play in the new Public Health movement, but we must have an independent watchdog keeping a close eye on the public health implications on such things as privatisation of water supplies, school meals and parts of the National Health Service and the introduction of a poll tax. Indeed we cannot get a new Public Health Alliance off the ground too soon! Privatisation is supposed to be about efficiency but, in my opinion, it really is about making financial profits. That is not an effective motive for improving standards of health or care (as shown in USA). The Public Health Alliance will seek to expose and make clear the relationships (and ethics) between interests of MPs and others in authority to forces which are antagonistic to health, such as the tobacco industry, alcohol industry and parts of food and pharmaceutical industry. Also requiring exposure are those health researchers who accept funding from the tobacco industry at the suggestion of the DHSS. In addition, it has proven useful to bring to the attention of investors who unwittingly support companies producing unhealthy products to this fact. Thus two years ago a survey of investors in the tobacco industry was carried out by Social Audit, the British Medical Association and Health Education Council. The results were published with great publicity. A year later a second survey revealed that almost all major investors who had connections with health or the churches had got rid of their tobacco shares. There are now a few Investment Trusts, like The Stewardship Unit Trust, which are successful financially, but which do not invest in tobacco, alcohol, arms or South Africa.

The new public health movement can also make understandable and human, health statistics which are a potent indicator of inequalities in health, of deprivation and disadvantage. This was borne out by the original Black Report in 1980 and several reports in 1987 such as 'The Health Divide: Inequalities in the 1980s' by Margaret Whitehead.

One example: the Black Report showed childhood fatal accidents to be five times more common in Social Class V compared with Social Class I. 'The Health Divide' showed the difference to be a factor of seven.

Other such reports published this year and showing similar trends were 'Investing in the Future' by the National Children's Bureau, and 'The Growing Divide' published by the Child Poverty Action Group.

Identifying areas of inequality and deprivation is fundamental to the cure. Thus, first diagnose – then treat. Furthermore, the cure is using existing resources in a deliberate and focused fashion, in other words, positive discrimination. Professor Alwyn Smith, immediate past President of the Faculty of Community Medicine, stated in a recent lecture at Green College, Oxford: 'The notion that inequalities in health call for directed innovative action is the central premise on which medical practice is based.' Also it was Robert Virchow, father of cellular pathology, who said. 'Physicians have always been the natural advocates of the poor', and Aristotle who said, 'Treat equals equally, and unequals unequally'.

All in all, I would identify inequalities and poverty as the main dangers to the public health. Given our present resources among the steps we can take are the following:

(1) The resources of Local Authority and the National Health Service must be combined and work together to achieve equality in health. They must together set targets based on WHO Health For All 2000. Such local co-operation between the National Health Service and Local Authority should be supplemented by bringing in local industry and voluntary organisations. My own wish is to see a greater involvement of the cooperative societies and the various women's voluntary organisations. And, very importantly, the churches. They must join in a social and religiously based alliance.

(2) The changes we need from Government are fundamental. These demand, firstly, a recognition that unemployment is harmful to mental and physical health. Secondly, the fundamental change that is required is a re-distribution of disposable income. Poverty is the underlying cancer explaining inequalities in health. This was the main recommendation of the Black Report. Small increases for the poor would significantly improve their health while comparable reductions for the rich would have little effect. The Chancellor of Exchequer and indeed the whole cabinet bear a heavy responsibility for health indeed.

(3) We in the health teaching and caring professions must combine with other professions such as the law and the clergy. Let me refer you to the 1984 Richard Dimbleby Lecture by the Right Reverend David Shepherd, Bishop of Liverpool. The title was 'The poverty which imprisons the spirit' and he was talking about material poverty. He shares the anger we must develop. He said: 'Twenty years in East and South East London; nine years in Liverpool. This baptism into the city leaves me with a feeling of indignation. I am angry when I see the sick human relationships which poverty spawns: depression, deference, fear, cynicism, jealousy and self-righteous blaming.'

To enable such changes, to be vigilant and to act as a resource for the public health in the United Kingdom, we need a focus and a banner. Edmund Burke said: 'When bad men combine, the good must associate, else they will fall one by one, an unpitied sacrifice in a contemptible struggle.' We need an engine for the new public health movement. We need an association of individuals and institutions. We need a Public Health Alliance!

Sir Donald Acheson, CMO, in his Duncan Memorial Lecture, 1986, said: 'The Secretary of State has said that he expects the new Health Education Authority to exercise 'the same sort of sturdy independence' as the HEC.' But at least one body with a fearless, totally independent voice outside Government should be available to pose the politically embarrassing question, or point to the awkward deficiency. Historically the Society of Medical Officers of Health in a corporate sense discharged this role. The weight of their authority was such that they forced important innovations on successive governments including the compulsory notification of infectious disease; and the provision of services for the control of tuberculosis.

Today this function is split between the Royal College of Physicians, the other Colleges, Government funded bodies like ASH and Alcohol Concern, the BMA and the College of Health, all of whom do good work. Is this splintering inevitable? Should the Faculty of Community Medicine try to take up the mantle of the Society of Medical Officers of Health? Or have we reached a time when an exclusively medical organisation cannot fit the bill and as Richard Smith has suggested we need a 'Public Health Alliance'!

This was launched in Birmingham in July 1987 at a two-day conference organised by Birmingham City Council, Lambeth Council, Health Rights and the Health Education Council and funded by the HEC.

The background to this Public Health Alliance initiative has been a growing interest in public health in the United Kingdom and other industrialised countries and within the World Health Organisation. Despite the resources invested and the progress made in health care, preventative medicine and environmental health, many people are not able to lead lives that are as healthy as they could be. It is increasingly recognised that there are many pre-requisites for health, including enough healthy food, safe air and water, decent housing and adequate education and income. Health education aimed at encouraging people to adopt healthy personal life-styles needs to be complemented by attention to the pre-requisites for health. The new interest in public health emphasises the environmental determinants of health and the important influence of all aspects of public policy on people's health.

In July 1986, a group of about 50 people with a keen interest in improving public health in the UK first met at the Health Education Council to consider the formation of a public health alliance to develop support for public health in the UK. The need for such support was apparent for several reasons:

- the health aspect of many policy decisions is either not considered or not given enough importance (e.g., in housing, unemployment or transport policy);

- there are some subjects (e.g., raising childhood immunisation rates) about which individuals and groups are concerned but where there is no comprehensivecampaign;

- campaigns on some issues (e.g., alcohol abuse) are making little or no progress;

- the most compelling reason for forming a new organisation is to provide a unique overview of all public health issues – healthy public policy, environmental health, illness and accident prevention, and mental and physical health promotion.

Objectives and organisation

No existing British organisation is already carrying out the work envisaged nor would one of the existing organisations be suitable for developing the comprehensive role that is needed (comparable in many ways to that of the Canadian or American Public Health Associations). Indeed, the case for the formation of a public health alliance in the UK has received strong support from the *British Medical Journal*. Keen interest has also been expressed by many individuals and organisations throughout the UK.

The Steering Group that was set up in 1986 to bring a Public Health Alliance into being has, after consultation, drawn up the following objectives and proposals for organisation:

(1) To provide a national focus for stimulating health promotion activities in the UK applying the WHO targets for Health For All by the year 2000 and the WHO principles of health promotion as expressed in the 1986 Ottawa Charter on Health Promotion. (The WHO targets, to which the UK government is a signatory, embrace six major themes: reducing inequalities in health: promoting health and preventing disease, stimulating community participation in health promotion and care; involving all sectors of government and society concerned with factors that influence health; giving greater emphasis to primary health care and encouraging international co-operation.)

(2) To identify and strengthen existing coalitions of organisations whose activities and interests relate to improving people's health and to identify and help initiate new coalitions where relevant.

(3) To provide resources to organisations to help research and practical activities which promote people's health. The Public Health Alliance would act as a 'clearing house' which would collect, hold and provide public-health information, thus avoiding duplication of effort by other organisations and enabling them to share resources and experience. In time, the Alliance might be able to provide financial resources, either directly or by seeking contributions from other sources.

(4) To provide a lead in research, documentation and practical initiatives which will stimulate a wider awareness and application of health promotion. The Alliance would, in the first instance, seek to publish reports and other information contributed by members and would want eventually to establish its own research unit. This would aim to produce studies on a wide range of public-health issues, including public policy.

Already about 300 individuals have joined as well as important organisations such as: Association of CHC's of England and Wales, Alcohol Concern, Action on Alcohol Abuse, Age Concern, London Food Commission, Lothian Regional Council, National Association of Health Authorities, Friends of the Earth, Scottish Association of Local Health Councils, and The Institute of Environmental Health Officers.

Many other organisations are considering association and support in committee, e.g. the Faculty of Community Medicine.

I am confident that the Public Health Alliance will survive.

References

1. Whitehead, M. (1987). The Health Divide: Inequalities in Health. London, Health Education Council.
2. Department of Health and Social Security. (1980). Inequalities in health. Report of a Research Working Group chaired by Sir Douglas Black. DHSS.
3. Townsend, P. & Davidson, N. (1982). Inequalities in health: the Black Report. Penguin.
4. World Health Organisation. (1985). Social justice and equity in health. A report from the social equity and health WHO meeting, Leeds.
5. Platt, S & Kreitman, N. (1984). Unemployment and parasuicide in Edinburgh 1968–82. *British Medical Journal,* 289, 1029–1032.
6. Marsh, G. N. & Channing, D.M. (1986). Deprivation and health in one general practice. *British Medical Journal* 292, 1173–1176.
7. Wandsworth, M.E.J. (1986). Serious illness in childhood and its association with later life achievement. In: Wilkinson, R.G. (ed.), *Class and Health: Research and Longitudinal Data.* London: Tavistock.
8. Illsley, R. (1986). Occupational class, selection and the production of inequalities in health. *Quarterly Journal of Sociological Affairs,* 2, 151–165.
9. Power, C., Fogelman, K. & Fox, A.J. (1986). Health and social mobility during the early years of life. National Child Development Study Working Paper No. 8, Social Statistics Research Unit, City University, London.
10. OPCS, (1986). General Household Survey for 1984. London: HMSO.
11. Cook, D.G., Bartley, M.J., Cummins, R.O. & Shaper, A.G. (1982). Health of unemployed middle-aged men in Great Britain. *Lancet,* i, 1290–1294.
12. Marmot, M.G., Shipley, M.J. & Rose, G. (1984). Inequalities in death – specific explanations of a general pattern? *Lancet,* i, 1003–1006.
13. Berkman, L.F. & Breslow, L. (1983). Health and Ways of Living: the Alameda County Study. Oxford University Press.
14. Thunhurst, C. (1985). Poverty and health in the City of Sheffield. Environmental Health Dept., Sheffield City Council.
15. Greater Glasgow Health Board. (1984). Ten Year Report 1974–1983: Glasgow, Greater Glasgow Health Board.
16. US Department of Health Education and Welfare. (1979). The Surgeon General's Report on Health Promotion and Disease Prevention. US Government Printing Office: Washington.
17. Lalonde, M. (1974). A New Perspective on the Health of Canadians. Ministry of Supply and Services: Canada.

Towards Healthy Public Policy in Food and Nutrition*

Public Health (1990), 104, 45–54. © The Society of Public Health, 1990.
Nancy Milio, PhD, Professor of Health Policy and Administration.
CB*7460 University of North Carolina, Chapel Hill, North Carolina
27599–7460, USA.

Here are the sources of needlessly high rates of disease, especially among disadvantaged people: poor diet, inactivity, inadequate hygienic habits, lack of coping skills, and generally imprudent lifestyles.[1,2] This was the judgement not of the latest health reports but of British and American authorities 150 years ago. They echoed the same widely held view that attempted to account for high levels of illness and death in Liverpool's outcasts during the time of William Henry Duncan (1805–1862), the first Medical Officer of Health (1847–1862).[3]

We in the human family view the world at any point in time by focusing on either figure or ground, person or context, object or environment. We do not perceive both at the same moment. As in Duncan's time, many people today continue to focus primarily on the individual and his or her habits or 'lifestyle' when defining health issues and the means to address them. Others, as did Duncan, are again focusing on the context, people's environment, which frames the array of options available to individuals and from which they, for good or ill health, choose the patterns that become their lifestyles.

Most people, as most organisations, including governments, most of the time make the choices that are easiest, closest to hand, most rewarding within their immediate context, 'they' ('the people'), just as 'we' ('the experts').

Duncan quickly (re)learned this lesson when, in one of his early efforts as Medical Officer of Health, he attempted to remove some 30,000 people from their quarters in 8,000 dank, airless, undrained cellars, leaving hundreds to live in the streets. They immediately returned to their hovels where at least they were less exposed to weather and danger, and had access to the cake and fruits that were often sold at the entrances to the cellars.[3] The people, in other words, chose the best they could among the miserable options available to them.

When later Duncan faced the onslaughts of a wave of impoverished famine victims from Ireland and a cholera epidemic, he learned further that 'environment' is not a closed context, but extends beyond local communities.

---

* The 6th Duncan Memorial Lecture presented at The University of Liverpool, PO Box 147, Liverpool L69 3BX.

What Duncan learned from these experiences, and from his earlier voluntary work in public clinics, as well as from his acquaintance with Chadwick's ideas, he spoke out about. At first, his audience was his medical peers, through lectures and journals. Soon it was politicians and local opinion leaders, through testimony, reports, public lectures and pamphlets. He took his case, in effect, to the gatekeepers of public discourse, to political and lay leaders, and translated his message – of the primacy for health of the environment and of the policies that shape that environment – into their languages and through the media available in that era. And when he was blocked by local authorities from instituting preventive policies to improve living conditions, he took his case to national authorities and won.

Today, in a far larger and more complex world, we can take lessons from Duncan's strategy and persistence, and encouragement from his successes, even though they were neither complete nor eternal. The advances he made, and the model he developed, one that became contagious throughout the United Kingdom, were not primarily the result of 'hard science' (the miasma theory was not sustainable) or of hardware. Improvements in the public's health were rather the result of 'soft data' – political rationales and persuasive public language – and social software ('groupware') – organisational action both public and private.

This is what today's move toward a new or renewed public health is about, and what in particular its cornerstone, 'healthy public policy' is about. In other words, as asserted in a recent unusual report on the state of the public health enterprise in the US by the national Institute of Medicine, 'Health is a political issue', requiring leaders to think and act strategically, taking into account social and political forces and policy sectors beyond conventional health services.[4]

To illustrate the effort toward creating an intersectoral approach to health policy in our time, a time in which we are acutely aware that 'everything is related to everything else', a time perhaps inspired by a beckoning new Century, I will focus on nutrition-health issues as a policy problem. I draw my remarks from recent research.[5]* In particular, I will sketch current policy environment and strategies that are being or could be pursued to move national food and nutrition policy forward – policy that requires cooperation among many policy sectors (e.g., agriculture, health, environment, education, communication, industry, trade, finance, planning), as well as involvement of commercial, voluntary and government, national and local groups.

The policy environment

The time is ripe for an intersectoral policy approach to nutrition. The policy climate is in readiness, and we know that policy works best when it is timely, when it can fuse with currents in the milieu and guide them in desirable and, in this case, healthier directions than might otherwise occur. Readiness is the precondition for effective policymaking. The signals of this readiness are many.

---

* Detailed references can be found in Milio, in press.

Policy ferment

It is fair to say that agricultural policy in every major nation is in ferment. The impetus comes from growing surpluses among the food-rich and deficits among the food-poor: protectionism and debt-ridden buyers; the imminence of open borders in the European Community, revision of its farm policy, and the inclusion of agriculture in GATT (General Agreement on Tariffs and Trade) negotiations.

There is also growing concern about technology-intensive abuse of the environment, documented by the World Commission on Environment and Development, and at least some acknowledgement, renewed from the early Seventies, that the food and nutrition problems among the food-rich are related to the problems of food-poor nations.

Less developed countries, such as Portugal as it enters the affluent milieu of the European Community, are giving policy attention to ways of avoiding the excess nutrition of their Northern partners. Portugal is seeking to forgo the North's overabundant, high fat, salty, refined diet, taking an intersectoral approach to what has been called 'primordial' (not just 'primary') prevention.

Legitimacy

In the health policy sector throughout the world, officials are now *accepting* the evidence that has been available for 30 years on the link between modern diets and chronic disease. The mammoth *Report on Nutrition and Health* (1988) by the US Surgeon General is only the most recent example. This belated but welcome attention may have been spurred by estimates that over 70% of US deaths are due to diet-related illness, as are about half of the premature deaths below age 65 among Europeans.[6] This implies greater costs for already costly medical care systems. Such cost-burdens are a persistent problem in almost every nation, for they often require resources that might otherwise go toward other national goals.

As a result, governments have been willing to support, from the early Seventies, large scale community intervention trials (as well as conventional clinical dietary studies, epidemiological surveys and animal experiments) to test whether calorie-controlled diets low in saturated fats, cholesterol, sugar, alcohol, and sodium and high in complex carbohydrates and fibre could reduce the risks of cardiovascular diseases, some cancers, dental and other diseases. The research shows, in countries as diverse as Finland, Belgium, New Zealand, and Australia, that efforts directed toward community-based organisations and governments could bring about programmes and policies to support dietary changes in populations and consequently reduce the risk of chronic disease.[7,8] One minimal result of the widely distributed findings has been the development of national dietary guidelines for a 'New Nutrition', from Norway to Japan, Canada to Brazil.

Changing populations

People are ready to hear a new nutrition-health message and to act on it – but not without guidance and incentives. The aging and increasingly well-educated, employed and affluent populations in the advanced industrial nations from West to East are becoming a source of political and economic support for initiating policy guidance for improved food quality and new options for consumption.

Their readiness is importantly related to demographic and social changes. An increasing share of the population are in the older ages and a declining share are youth. Family and household arrangements are being altered by declining marriage rates, later marriage, more divorces, fewer children per couple, wider entry into the world of paid work by women and youth, and more 'singles' and two-career couples.

Dietary changes

These overall shifts in living arrangements and increases in disposable income, especially among women, youth, and elders suggest that what people *need* to eat (e.g. children's milk vs. an employee's snack or lunch), what they can afford to buy (e.g. low cost staple commodities vs. costlier prepared or restaurant foods), and what they *prefer* (e.g. family 'leftovers' vs. 'slimming' foods) can be expected to continue to alter typical dietary patterns, and nutrition and health as well. This demographic aspect of the social texture is then relevant for policy design and strategic action.

The changes in dietary patterns that have occurred in recent decades, contributing to modern health problems among food-rich populations, also contain suggestive elements of a potentially more healthful direction.

As a fairly typical example of both the problems and promise of current dietary trends, US adults, 19–50 years, in the mid-Eighties consumed about 37% of their daily food energy in fats including 13% from saturated fats. Carbohydrates contributed about 46% of calories, often in refined and sugared products (20%), the remaining share derived from relatively large amounts of protein (18%) and alcohol (3%). This meant that over 80% ate less than the recommended amounts of fibre (20–30 gm), more than 'prudent' levels of fat (i.e. 30%) and saturated fat (i.e. 10%), and almost half at too much cholesterol (i.e. over 300 mg), resulting in serum cholesterol levels that placed 26% of employees at risk for coronary heart disease.

Overall food energy for all persons (aged 1–74) was in excess of need on average, which along with increasing sedentary living and alcohol consumption since the mid-Seventies, resulted in growing shares of obese children, adolescents, and adults (over 25% based on ideal, long-life weight in the mid-Eighties), including 26% of employed people. This represents increases in the prevalence of obesity of 54% among adults and of 98% among 6–11 year olds between 1965–80, based on National Centre for Health Statistics data.

In general, women and elders, who are mainly women, have food patterns and body weights closer to the dietary guidelines than men or younger people through eating less meat and more fish, cereals, and fresh produce.

Eating sites

Given the social facts of more working and independent adults and fewer children, these nutrient trends require that policy-relevant questions be asked about *who* is buying and using which foods and *where* they are eating.

Recent data show, for example, that within the long term drop in dairy product consumption per capita, cheese use in the US doubled in the last 20 years, but mainly through away-from-home eating habits and processed foods, such as pizza (62% of cheese consumption), rather than home use (38%) where it is declining. Whole milk is used less per person because of fewer babies, and is being replaced by low-fat milk (among weight-conscious workers). While butter consumption is steady overall, it has dropped in home use, 70% of it now consumed ('hidden') in processed foods. And half of all fats are now eaten in processed foods. These patterns suggest areas that nutrition policy could effectively address, such as food processing and food services.

Money matters

Contrary to the assumptions of some observers, changes in food consumption most closely parallel variations in prices and income, which for example, account for about 95% of the changes in dairy product trends. And these economic influences are related to the social patterns just noted. For example, in contrast to one-earner families, single households in the US spend almost twice as much of their food dollar (60%) away from home; and career couples, compared to similar ones with children, spend 50% more away from home, less on dairy products, and more on 'convenience', time-saving home meals.

In effect, the relatively new economics-related independent living arrangements (including independent elderly women, living on public or private pensions), increasingly 'expose' new demographic groups to non-traditional nutritional options. These include, as suggested above, more cheese, butter, saturated vegetable oils, sodium, and sweeteners that are relatively more available in restaurants, fast food, processed and 'convenience' products than are used at home. At the same time, the larger demographic share of elders and women, given their comparatively favourable nutritional patterns, also favourably affect consumption trends. These trends will accelerate during the 1990s.

Nutritional nirvana?

Does this mean we are 'automatically' heading toward nutritional nirvana? Unfortunately, the more favourable nutrient intake among women and elders may not be biologically significant. For example, only a third of US women take less than the recommended maximum of 35% of calories from fat, only 12% fall below the stricter 30% standard, and just 10% eat less than 10% of food energy from saturated fat. Similarly, although older people eat less fat, their P/S ration (0.36) is not better than that for the total population, indicating that the composition of their fat intake does not improve.

Public information

Is more dietary information the answer? The evidence suggests that in itself, whether derived from nutritional education or advertising, it is not enough to significantly effect healthy changes in overall population food patterns. Commercial promotion, for example, has slowed but not stopped the decline in home use of fluid milk and cheese.

The effects of health and nutrition information and attitudes are even more nebulous. If, for example, knowledge of the 'New Nutrition' were the basis for the increase in low-fat milk products, it does not account for the more rapid growth in consumption of relatively high saturated fat cheeses, which more likely is related to *where* Americans eat. Further, in spite of the purported awareness and interest of Americans in 'healthy lifestyles' portrayed by the mass media and commercial advertisers, adults (20–74 years), as noted, are more obese, more sedentary and drink more alcohol than a decade ago.

Americans, however, are not sufficiently knowledgeable about nutrition. About 75% do not know the major diet-health links and cannot name low fat, low sodium, high fibre, and high calorie foods. And even when highly knowledgeable people, in a major controlled trial, reported health-related changes in food buying and preparation, those changes were not large enough to affect local supermarket sales of New Nutrition foods. Further, only a fourth or less of supermarket (blue-collar) shoppers are concerned about fats or prepare meals in ways to reduce it.

New immigrants

One source of influence that could affect food patterns in favour of the New Nutrition, is the growth of ethnic minorities from the Mediterranean, the East, and Latin America within the US and in other Western industrialised countries. To the extent that immigrants preserve their traditional cuisines and create both a demand for and supply of them, they will be a force toward higher fibre, lower fat, less processed food patterns. Again, policy attention here, in support of healthy food markets and eating places, could foster not only the New Nutrition but small business and local community development as well.

Market manoeuvres

Complementing the readiness of the political and social climate for a New Nutrition, the 'market' also stands poised. This is true at least with respect to capturing 'upscale' customers, those with a lifestyle that seeks convenient and attractive, slimming, away-from-home foods, without too much regard to price.

This prospect has not been lost on the producers of high-fat, high-sugar products or those with high fibre and fresh foods. They tend to 'position' their advertising claims between the Scylla of nutrition science and the Charybdis of 'truth in advertising' regulations, often leading the consumer on a confusing and wayward journey to a 'healthy' diet. For example, the US beef industry's claim to low-fat products are based on 2–3 oz servings – an unlikely amount for most meat eaters – attractively, but dubiously pictured as *three* slices of braised rare beef.[9, 10]

The class chasm

A final policy-relevant dimension of the environment, one that cuts across all of these others – nutrients, health risks, and food; gender, age, and ethnicity; living arrangements and employment; food processing and pricing; meal sites, selection, and preparation; information and food availability – is the persistent and sometimes widening socioeconomic gap favouring the favoured. This is a poorly-addressed fact of social life in both the UK and the USA. Over the last decade the disparities have been growing among rich and poor in diet-related low birthweight babies and infant mortality, dietary risk factors, and diet-related disease and deaths.[11–14]

Left to the marketplace, both the New Nutrition and those groups with less access to the market, are likely to be limited to profitable products available according to sales peaks, while offered a sustained assortment of lesser-priced, less healthful choices.[15]

Policy action

Given this general atmosphere existing in many countries – where farm and trade policies are in ferment, where there is wide awareness of diet-health links and of ever-rising medical costs, and where lifestyles and markets are changing – many policymakers have seen political value in moving forward on nutrition issues. Accordingly, some countries and regions have gone further than simply providing public dietary information. They have established a new generation of community demonstrations and/or established new bodies for a New Nutrition, potential milestones in the development of intersectoral nutrition policies.

These have been supported not only or even mainly by the health sector, but also by agriculture and industry.

New projects

What is unique about the Eighties' community projects is that they address not only the consumer (demand) – persuading or informing individuals about healthy food choices. They also address food supply issues, requiring involvement of producers, processors, marketers, and retailers. Some have the explicit intent to influence national policymaking.

Projects in Finland, Wales, Stockholm, Melbourne, and Liverpool have taken lessons from the successful North Karelia experiment. There, people's behaviour changed in healthful ways, not by an increase in their dietary knowledge (which did not occur) but because their environments were changed in ways that made healthy choices more available and acceptable.

Yet even these sophisticated projects have met impasses when economic incentives, based on national government policies, have made the making of healthier choices in food supply by *industry* harder than holding to current practices.[16, 17] A healthy food and nutrition policy would make such *industry* choices 'easier', i.e., less risky to their profit margin.

New bodies

Thus several countries, taking the policy implications of these food and nutrition projects – which demonstrate both the strength of an integrated supply-demand approach and the limits of solely localised efforts – have established, pre-policy bodies intended to address the scope of intersectoral policy issues for a New Nutrition.

In Northern Europe alone, for example, Finland set up a multi-member ministerial board, chaired by Agriculture, intended to design a food and nutrition policy by 1990; a similar body was formed in the Ministry of Health in Denmark; and in the Netherlands and Ireland bureaus were established independent of the ministries.

These policy-relevant bodies vary widely in composition and resources. Most are advisory, some are led by health professionals, others by political leaders from outside or within the health sector. Some attempt to address the full scope of policy issues. And they move at different speeds, using informational rather than economic or political tools.

Yet their very existence represents the legitimising and renewal of efforts to 'marry agriculture and health' first proclaimed by the League of Nations in the 1930s. Most of these groups are aware of and to some extent have been influenced by Norway's well-known 1975 intersectoral food and nutrition policy.

As a further indication of widespread recognition of the importance of nutrition policy, WHO set up a Nutrition office to support policy development among European nations in 1984.

The next step

Taken together, the prevailing social climate and political activity suggest a broad consensus among food-rich countries on the general direction for healthful dietary changes, and sufficient internal political support to publicly finance public nutrition education, a few community-based projects, and incipient forms of strategic apparatus to help focus attention on nutrition policy development.

But can the new pre-policy machinery actually produce effective food and nutrition policy? The answer depends on whether and how policymakers face three major policy issues, namely, the choice of policy goals and of policy instruments, and the strategic capacity to implement them.

The issues

The first issue concerns the goal and scope of policy, principally the degree and quality of dietary fat reduction. Where scientific criteria suggest a 30% limit, mainly by lowering animal and saturated vegetable fats to 10% of energy intake, political criteria may dictate a higher (e.g., 35%) or unspecified limit or a less specific focus on animal fats. Here the main constraint involves the vast economic and political influence of multinational industries engaged in not only dairy and beef, soy and feed grain production and trade but also the manufacture of large-scale farm equipment, fertilisers, and chemicals. Thus, the scope of food and nutrition policy could encompass, as in Norway, not only diet and health but also farm and food production and marketing, rural development and job creation, environmental conservation, and international aid and trade. The issue is whether policy intent is to influence supply and/or demand.

A second issue concerns the instruments the policy will employ. Will they be the politically and economically less risky tools of information, education, research and evaluation? Or will they be strengthened by more powerful measures for creating structural changes, such as revised subsidies and pricing, production controls, development and marketing support, and regulation of food composition and advertising?

A third major issue centres on the design of a strategic capacity (an organisational 'policykeeper') that can promote policy adoption and, once adopted, transform it into social reality.[5] This involves strategic apparatus, strategic planning, and the provision of political and economic resources to act effectively. Too many social policies have mandates for implementation without the co-requisite means to do so.

Strategy

The purpose of strategic apparatus for nutrition policy is to get nutrition-health issues on the agendas of relevant policy sectors and organisations, and collaborate with them on policy options that are more healthful for the population and for disadvantaged groups than might otherwise be. To be effective, these efforts must be informed by astute views of ongoing changes in the national and international climate of the sort I have outlined. Some of the essential ingredients for a strategic capacity which, in effect, can make an intersectoral food and nutrition policy feasible in a particular context, are suggested by the degrees of 'success' or 'failure' of nations that have led the way, most notably Norway with over a decade of experience.[5]

Accordingly, the 1980s' generation of New Nutrition bodies would do well to adopt a strategic stance. They should begin to *monitor selected aspects* of their environment and of the organisations whose cooperation they need. These include international currents, such as relevant actions by global centres of trade, prospects for world food security, and negotiations within the European Community, as well as national changes, including media depictions of nutrition issues and public perceptions of them. Further, the target organisations whose support they need should be identified and information obtained on their priorities, policy preferences, and sources of financial and constituency support in order to negotiate effectively with them.

The policykeeping groups must then be capable of assessing and drawing from its information base the *implications for strategic planning*. This includes defining or redefining (i.e., 'translating') the nutrition-health problem in terms that link it meaningfully to other economic and political issues that already are priorities for policymakers and their constituencies, the media, professionals and public. These might include rural unemployment, environmental protection, quality of life, social equity, rising health care costs and fiscal deficits. They should also outline tactical options for action to reach targeted policy leaders and other public and private commercial and non-profit groups. Beyond this, the timing of action, negotiating rationales and incentives should be prepared for use with both potential allies and competitor groups, as well as appropriate public communications.

Incentives, for example, that can induce groups to undertake supportive advocacy action or make shifts in their products or services, include helping protect them from significant economic, budgetary or 'image'-related risks. These could involve assistance with or provision of such in-kind resources as training and materials, public opinion, marketing, and other survey data and analyses, promotion, endorsements and technical assistance. Further inducements might be the prospects for publicity and enhanced credibility by involvement in nutrition, health, and quality-of-life issues and actions, which in turn could have political or economic value to the cooperating governmental or private target group.

For New Nutrition bodies to sustain such an effort clearly requires strategic *capacity-building resources* – funds, committed leadership, legitimacy, technical expertise, access to information and to high level policymakers. Most of the new bodies do not have this capacity-base. Without it, they face heavy constraints.

While nothing can fully substitute for an adequate and sustainable resource base, these organs can do some reprioritising of the resources they already have. To the extent that they are restricted to using only information (rather than economic or regulatory) instruments, they should go beyond simply offering sound consumer dietary information or analyses of 'hard' epidemiological or clinical data. Rather, they can direct their 'soft' data toward decision-makers, national and local, to persuade, activate, and mobilise them to use their own resources to support policy development.

They would in effect use a support-building information strategy. This means one that focuses on new audiences – the gatekeepers to public discourse: political and organisational leaders and media editors – and people-as-citizens or constituents, using new types of information (e.g., health-related political rather than personal types) and new channels (e.g., media, organisational, and political rather than counselling and classrooms).[5]

Another adjustable resource, time, should be allocated to cultivate and sustain ties with groups potentially affected by policy changes, including political parties and factions, legislative and bureaucratic units, voluntary and commercial groups, as well as the news media. Further, supportive and collaborative ties should be formed with a variety of community groups relevant to health development. Capacity-building may extend to strengthening their abilities to participate effectively in local health development through organisational support services such as collaborative training and technical assistance.

The New Nutrition bodies, whether government-appointed or self-proclaimed, can, in other words, be assertive, in spite of ever-present resource constraints.

The food-poor

In the areas of food, nutrition and health, some policymakers, analysts, and concerned groups are coming to recognise that the solution to the health and economic problems of overnutrition in food-rich countries and populations is related to the solution of undernutrition in food-poor nations and peoples and to the emerging chronic disease patterns threatening developing countries.

The food-rich are in a position to support, for example, multisectoral policy machinery among the food-poor, and research and development of organisational methods and programmes that create sustainable labour-intensive, farm-food systems – especially those that build women's income-earning capacity and food production and marketing abilities.

Beyond this change in food aid policy, the food-rich nations could ease their own nutrition-health problems by creating national sustainable agricultures, including policy-guided shifts in the mix as well as amount of the food supply, in farm and food subsidies, and in trade practices.

The New Nutrition bodies, if they joined in collective action, could become vehicles for strengthening the health and nutrition message in international and national policy arenas. Together the European bodies could influence national and Continental agricultural and food policies that must in any case change as the European Community moves towards its open-border goals. Similarly, they could strengthen the efforts of multilateral organisations concerned with world food security.

Conclusion

A chronic nutrition-health problem persists in virtually every nation: too much food for some and too little for others, and not the healthiest mix for either. At bottom the solution depends on whether the presumed 'invisible hand' of the market or an informed public voice expressed through public policy and collective action can best improve the prospects for health. The adherents of the (alleged) free market approach have captured the public space for some years. It is time for another message to be heard and enacted. The environment is ready, but better health does not just 'happen'. It requires committed, organised leadership and action to shape the *possibilities* into healthier directions for all and not just some of us.

References

1. Rosenburg, C. (1962). *The cholera years: The United States in 1832, 1849 and 1866*. Chicago: University of Chicago Press.
2. Morris, R. (1976). *Cholera, 1832*. London: Holmes and Meier.
3. Chave, S.P. (1984). The Duncan memorial lecture: Duncan of Liverpool – and some lessons for today. *Community Medicine*, 6, 61–71.

4. Institute of Medicine (1988). *The future of public health.* Washington, DC: Academy of Sciences Press.

5. Milio, N. (in press). *Nutrition policy for food-rich   countries.* Baltimore: Johns Hopkins University Press.

6. Nutrition Unit. (1986). *Healthy nutrition: Preventing nutrition-related diseases in Europe.* Copenhagen: World Health Organisation.

7. Puska, P. (1986). *Comprehensive cardiovascular control   programmes in Europe: Description and experiences of the WHO/Euro coordinated programme.* Puska, B. (ed.). Copenhagen: World Health Organisation.

8. Casswell, S. (1986). *Evaluation of the community action project on alcohol.* Alcohol Research Unit. New Zealand: University of Auckland.

9. Beef Industry Council (1987). *Meatstyles.* Chicago.

10. Keys, A., et al. (1988). Effect of dietary stearic acid on plasma cholesterol level. *New England Journal of Medicine,* 319, 1089.

11. Marmot, M. & McDonnell, M. (1986). Mortality decline and widening social inequalities. *Lancet,* ii, 274–276.

12. Scott-Samuel, A. & Blackburn, P. (1988). Crossing the health divide – mortality attributable to social inequality in Great Britain. *Health promotion,* 2, 243–245.

13. Wing, S., *et al.* (1987). Changing association between community occupational structure and ischemic heart disease mortality in the United States. *Lancet,* ii, 1067–70.

14. National Commission to Prevent Infant Mortality (1988). *Death before life: The tragedy of infant mortality.* Washington, DC: The Commission.

15. Levine, J. (1986). Hearts and minds: The politics of diet and heart disease. In: *Consuming Fears* Sapolsky, R. (ed.), p. 42- 79, New York: Basic Books.

16. Milio, N. (1986). *Promoting health through public policy* (softback edition). Ottawa: Canadian Public Health Association.

17. Milio, N. (1986). Health and the media – an uneasy relationship. *Community Health Studies,* 10, 419–422.

Food Policy and Public Health

Public Health (1992), 106, 91–125. ©The Society of Public Health, 1992.
7th Duncan Memorial Lecture University of Liverpool, November 1989.
T. Lang PhD. (Director, London Food Commission 1984–1990);
Director, Parents for Safe Food, c/o National Food Alliance, 102
Gloucester Place, London W1H 3DA.

Introduction

I feel honoured to have been chosen to lecture to you tonight for three reasons. First, Duncan was someone who put public health action before other considerations – a timely reminder for us given the sometimes dire position of public health in Britain today. Second, I am honoured as a representative of the voluntary sector to speak in the memory of such a distinguished medical pioneer.

Third, lecturers often try to summon up links with their venue, but actually mine are fairly close. My great grandparents were from Liverpool, and one of my relatives, just recently died – otherwise we would have invited her – was England's one and only woman chief public analyst. Public analysts are the unsung heroes and, in my cousin twice removed's case, heroine of the UK food system. Their profession came to eminence in that great battle for the hearts and minds of the country over food adulteration in the mid-nineteenth century. The great institutional legacy of that fight is the local authority responsibility for what we today call Environmental Health, Trading Standards and Public Analysis.

I remind you of these three wings of the 'old' public health movement – medical, local authority and voluntary – because my experience in the 1980s has taught me that the 'new' public health movement works most effectively, whether as service provider or lobby or consciousness moulder, if all three wings work together. The state of food and food policy in Britain today illustrates the challenge we all face. Our responsibility is awesome. The forces we face are better funded, often better prepared, but rarely have better arguments. As a footsoldier in this tussle, I often find the work of our predecessors such as Duncan inspiring and supportive.

In this paper I want to do three things:

1. Stand back and review the food and public health scene at the end of the 1980s.

2. Pick out key issues in food policy as I see them.

3. Look ahead to the 1990s and sketch tension points that all of us in public health and food policy will inevitably be drawn into in the 1990s.

The 1980s have been hard times for a public health perspective in the UK. There are, nevertheless, some strategic possibilities whereby those of us who want to improve food availability, information, education, choice and enjoyment for all can pursue those honourable ends. Public culture is schizophrenic, both for and against public health, aware of private responsibility but supporting public provision, too. Food, although the example *par excellence* of an individual responsibility (we have to lift the fork into our own mouth after childhood!) is none the less a public responsibility, for who can grow, distribute, process and cater all their food in today's world? The separation of individual from the land fundamentally limits private responsibility. That is why the Government was so surprised that its role in the recent food scandals earned it opprobrium from all sides of the health spectrum. However rich, influential, powerful you are, you cannot have total control over your food. In this respect, the modern food and public health movement and the public have merely re-educated each other. Now it is time to take stock about what needs to change.

Time to review

At the end of the 1980s we are at a crucial moment for reviewing the whole of the post-war food revolution. In the immediate post-war period food policy in the UK and Europe was dominated by concern to deal with the problems of scarcity and post-war reconstruction. With the 1947 Agriculture Act, the United Kingdom food policy reversed the approach of the pre-war period: *laissez-faire* in agriculture at home and buying from colonies or abroad – the policy of imperial preference.[1]

Throughout Europe, ravaged by the Second World War, food policies were put in place which strongly emphasised the need to support agricultural systems. Diverse though these were between countries, there were common themes: to feed people, to rebuild primary production and to bolster middle Europe threatened by the Cold War. The ground was set for the problems of food policy as we understand them today.[2] The Common Agricultural Policy in all its contradictory glory was born.

Today public interest and medical interest in food as public health food issues are once more at a high level. It is said often that these are the concerns of affluence, and that we should never forget the problems of scarcity. I agree. Nevertheless we must also recognise that in the post-war period, there has also been a down-side to the food revolution.

From the consumers' point of view, the post-war period has seen a jump out of the frying pan of scarcity into the fire of environmental and public health problems which are and were avoidable. Within the corridors of Whitehall, the interests of production have triumphed over health and the environment.

The above assessment is not intended as a simplistic attack on production. Consumers need food to be produced! The questions now being addressed to the food producers by the consumer, public health and environment movements alike are not *whether* to produce, but *how*, with what impact on health, quality and environment? The opportunity to pose these questions comes in part from seeing the down-side of modern food production methods, and in part from the absence of scarcity. We need not be ashamed of this luxury.

The irony is that, just as we are relearning the need for an integrated, balanced food policy in Europe, the focus of decision making within Europe is shifting from national states to international states. The removal of barriers to trade by the end of 1992 places both a threat and a challenge to consumers and public health interests within Europe. Unless we create better trans-national understanding and communality of perspective, we will have little chance of righting the imbalances of the post-war food policy. If we are serious about improving food policy throughout Europe, we must understand better the role of the state. The New Right have been particularly interested in this issue.[3,4]

Today in our nation-states we have essentially 1950s structures of food decision making, making complex decisions for the 21st century. There must be reform of both the Ministry of Agriculture, Fisheries and Food regarding our food policy. One without the other would be self-defeating. So far, despite massive pressure, reform of the state structures which oversee food and agriculture has been minuscule and stuttering. More energy has been expended by Government into resisting European harmonisation than into positive proposals.

In Europe, reform is being driven by the self-imposed 1992 schedule and the Single European Act, 1985, signed by the Government. However much it may protest, the UK is locked into a European schedule. The timetable is determining policy outcomes. Around 100 food-related Directives (laws) are due to be pushed into law by 1993. These will affect food ingredients, quality, information, labelling, inspection and hygiene, to name but a few. Hence the growing concern in the consumer movement to argue for more open debate, more 'transparency', more accountability.[5]

The consumer movement's argument is that, if national compositional standards are being removed in the interests of removal of barriers to trade, consumers deserve some improvement in the food policy process. So far there is little sign of a quantum leap on this score.

These issues of democracy, openness, standards, quality and health or environmental impact are not just abstract or academic challenges limited to Europe.

The current Uruguay Round of the General Agreement on Tariffs and Trade (GATT) – originally planned to be completed by the end of 1990 – will set the terms and conditions for the entire world agricultural and food commodity trade. The issues of standards, public health, consumer protection and environmental protection have taken a very low priority in the process of the Uruguay Round. There has been an extraordinary obsession in GATT with the issue of prices, subsidies and protectionism. There is more to food than price.

Whether we look at food policy from a perspective of GATT, 1992, or the UK, the case for change cries out. Public health and environmental protection receive far lower priority within the institutional decision-making process than do the interests of trade. This poses a direct challenge to proponents of a public health perspective on food. If we can no longer talk of national food policies, how do we organise, lobby and represent the public health case in new and distant fora of decision making? Some give a cynical, chauvinist and Little England response to the question. I urge you not to. Already consumer groups such as Consumers in the European Community Group, based in London, are actively tackling the structural questions.[6,7]

Vital matters will be decided in the coming period. Just when we are winning the battle for the minds if not yet the hearts of the British over issues such as the need to cut down intake of saturated fats to cut down our lamentable rate of coronary heart disease, our power to influence decisions gently floats over the Channel and Atlantic. The nutritional consensus has it that the southern or Mediterranean diet is significantly healthier than the diet of overprocessed, relatively high in saturated fat foods in the northern European diet. So will the removal of barriers to trade lead to southern Europe being swamped by the highly powerful and market-hungry northern European food conglomerates? Will 1992 be just a trade jamboree or can, even at this late stage, the public health interest triumph? Our responsibility in this respect to future generations is awesome. The possibility of a health-conscious Europe-wide food policy hangs in the balance.

The return of public debate about food policy

In the UK, as with many other countries world-wide, a public interest perspective on food policy has been driven initially by nutritional concerns, especially over coronary heart disease and food-related cancers.[8] It is clear that food policy is more than nutrition policy. To put it differently, a nutrition policy does not resolve the problems that are manifestly real in food policy.

Most starkly we can see the connection between nutrition and food policy when we look at the widening gap between developing countries' food trade balances and those of the industrial countries. This is the underpinning of mass starvation (Figure 1). It is no wonder that food policy becomes such a sensitive and at times emotional issue.

In Britain, critics of our food system are sometimes accused of perpetrating a media hype. UK food is fine, its defenders argue, or was until the critics came along. This thesis should be scrutinised.

Take food poisoning. If we look at the figures on salmonella food poisoning we find that they were rising steeply well before the story hit the media in late 1988 (see Figure 2, 'Food Poisoning: The Chicken Comes Home to Roost').

Or take coronary heart disease. It is well known that the figures on coronary heart disease were grounds for concern well before the National Advisory Committee on Nutrition Education (NACNE) scandal hit the headlines in 1983–84.[9] NACNE argued that the UK diet needed to reduce its fat intake: a fairly incontrovertible argument, but the report was held up from publication until leaked. Still today around 180,000 deaths per year occur in the United Kingdom due to coronary heart disease, which costs the National Health Service approximately £0.5 billion a year to treat. And that sum takes no account of

Developing countries' food balance turns negative

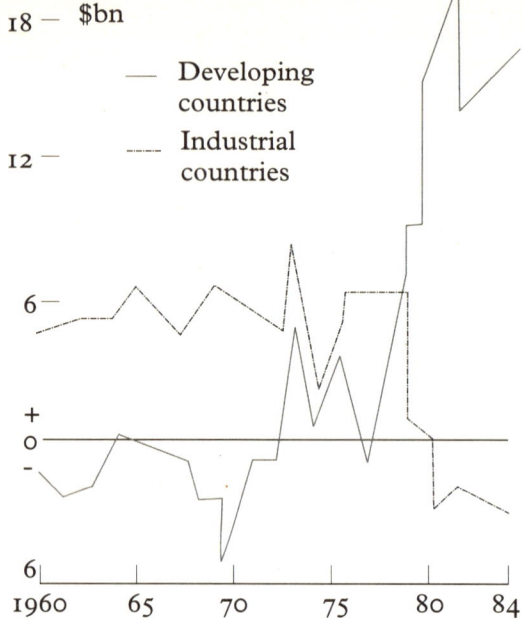

18 — $bn

—— Developing
countries

---- Industrial
countries

12 —

6 —

+
0
-

6

1960   65   70   75   80   84

Figure 1: Developing countries' food balance turns negative
Source: Leighton Morris/*Financial Times*

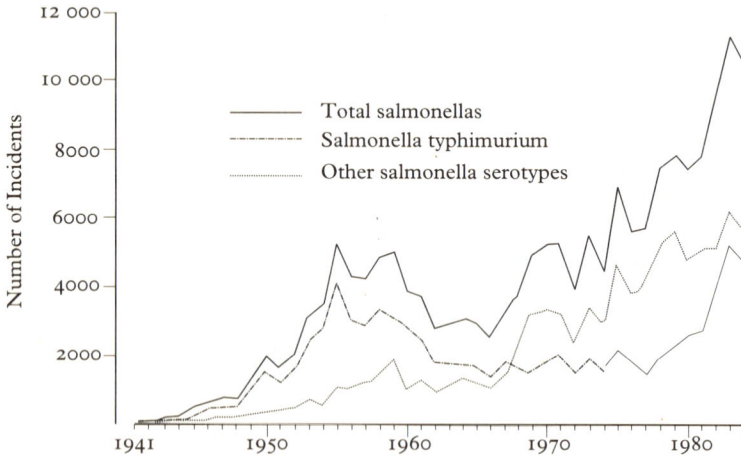

—— Total salmonellas
---- Salmonella typhimurium
.... Other salmonella serotypes

12 000
10 000
8000
6000
4000
2000

Number of Incidents

1941   1950   1960   1970   1980

Salmonellosis: England and Wales, 1941–84
(Source: Communicable Disease Surveillance Centre)

Figure 2: Food poisoning: the chicken comes home to roost.

the costs of unwaged family support, the human suffering, the lost working days and the reduction of human potential.

What is this term food policy?

Food policy may be defined as the aims and decisions which affect who eats what, when, where, how, on what terms and with what effect on health, environment, consumer choice.[10] Part of the UK's food policy crisis has been that our food policy is sometimes uncoordinated between the relevant key Ministries, notably the Department of Health and the Ministry of Agriculture, Fisheries and Food. We have seen this in the way in which the salmonella in eggs affair, which dominated the headlines between November 1988 and February 1989, and the listeria affair of 1989 were dealt with.

In this lack of coordination, Britain is not alone. Most advanced industrialised countries that I have visited appear to have a failure of proper coordination between the key food-related Ministries. Some are better than others. Poor structural coordination leads to poor policy coordination. Health policy goes in one direction, trade another, education another and so on. No wonder public food culture is schizophrenic, as I termed it earlier. We get at best divergent and at worst contradictory messages. It would help if Government tried to make its own food policy role explicit rather than implicit. And it would help all of us if we tackled all of the food policy jigsaw, and not just a few bits at a time. It is just as much of a mistake to see food policy as primarily an issue of food microbiological safety as to see it as primarily an issue of nutrition. It is both and much, much more.

A short account of UK food policy history
The debate about food policy is not new. In the UK in the eighteenth and nineteenth centuries, food quality and trading standards were major public issues, mainly because food was so flagrantly and often adulterated.

The nineteenth century anti-adulteration movement, as it was known, became a major force in changing British laws and in arguing the need for public health, preventive and protective measures. In the mid-nineteenth century modern food science, particularly chemistry, developed with independent-minded chemists and scientists, often gentlemen, helping to expose rampant food adulteration.[11]

The food industry of the time split between those who wanted to resist the predations and inquisitions of these interventionists, and those who recognised that by having tougher standards competition between the food companies could benefit those who held those tougher standards.

With new, strong food legislation, first in 1860 and then in 1875, the UK's food law structure, essentially still there, was in place. The key phrase in the 1984 Food Act, which held that food should be of the 'nature, quality and substance demanded', derives from the 1875 Act. It echoes the demands of the anti-adulteration movement. The phrase indicates a delicate balance between controls on the nature of production and the demands of the recipient of the food. Food should be wholesome, safe and what the customer ordered and envisaged. The emphasis, you note, is upon the consumer's demand to be pre-eminent. One of the good things that is happening today is a re-opening of debate within food science about who and what ends it serves.[12]

From the mid-nineteenth century to the early twentieth century in the UK, key elements in food policy debate were over free trade and protectionism and the consolidation of controls on adulteration. In the context of 1992, GATT and the global restructuring of the food economy, these debates urgently demand our attention. There is much to learn, for example about who gains and who loses from cheap food, from that period.

The trade and protectionism debate essentially was linked to the rise of Britain as a colonial empire. Should the UK be a manufacturing nation, fed by colonies providing cheap food? Should starvation be resolved by exporting surplus population to the colonies? Should preference in imports go to foods (and other commodities) derived from the empire? Should the United Kingdom's farming be left quietly to rot? These were the kinds of questions over which politicians and a wider public debated.[13]

The debates are well documented and need not be further amplified here, except to say that echoes of these debates are once more with us in the late twentieth century.[14] One need think only of the negotiations at an international level over the subsidies in world food trade – the General Agreement on Tariffs and Trade, above all – to make the point. Consider also the concern about the level of farm support within Europe compared to say Australia or the United States or to areas of the Third World.

The second major theme in early twentieth century food policy has less resonance to most food policy commentators today, which is a shame. The second theme was about who should monitor and audit the standards put into place by the anti-adulteration movement. There is little point promising better standards if there is no auditing and inspection for health and for value. A loaf should be a loaf. Food should be as the consumer 'demanded'. It should not make them ill.

The people given the task of this monitoring – for reasons which would have been familiar to Dr Duncan – were under local authority control. A tension between Central State and the Ministry, on the one hand, and the local state, the Borough or City or County, on the other, was in place. Today this is all being subtly redefined. Food law is more centralised, more deregulated, more 'scientised' (handed over to professionally defined experts) and less locally accountable.

My own view is that this tendency has helped create the conditions for the consumer backlash of the late 1980s. Thousands of new products or processes come to market every year. Local, let alone central state monitoring can hardly keep up, let alone pre-empt difficulties. Local control and inspection has little room to act as a counter-weight. Too much has relied upon trust in brands. 'Store X and Y must be alright.'

Social policy meets food policy

By the early twentieth century concern about food adulteration was taking second place to what we now call welfare concerns. Concern about poverty and its impact on food is nothing new. What do the poor eat? Is it bad for the national interest? From Engels to Booth, Mayhew and Rowntree, how the poor fed or failed to feed themselves was a critical issue.[15]

Enquiry after enquiry made by liberal welfare reformers and others with less liberal motives showed that there were serious problems in the working class and particularly the non-working class with regard to how food was cooked; the skills; the level of understanding about food management; the price and availability of food. The domestic science movement was one response. This argued that middle-class women should be trained in how to manage their food budgets efficiently. Their improved skills would act as a reservoir for training working people – particularly through domestic science. With the decline in domestic servants between the wars, domestic science was forced to change, as it has done again since the last war.

Another response to the welfare questions was the welfare food reform movement. This essentially took place in Britain in the guise of a number of piecemeal reforms. The Education (Provision of Meals) Act of 1906 gave power to the Treasury to levy a halfpenny rate to provide school meals for school-children. This Act came out of the liberal movement anxious to dissipate the growing and powerful working-class movement. It accompanied many humanitarian reforms such as national insurance, improved national housing and some occupational ill-health prevention measures.[16]

Most popularly, these liberal welfare reforms are associated with the 'shock' in the bastions of British society about the state of recruits for the Boer War. In fact the origin of these liberal welfare reforms goes back further than just the state of health of war recruits.

Throughout the early twentieth century we find reports into the state of factories, and a persistent theme that British industry and manufacturing could not possibly cope with the demands of international (particularly German) competition if it treated its labour force so disrespectfully. One only need remember the debate around the 1870 Education Act in which fear of being left behind by a better trained and educated Germany dominated, to make the point. Titmuss and particularly F. le Gros Clarke had their fingers on this debate. Again, their thoughts are well worth re-reading.[17]

There was also more than an element of political opportunism in reforms such as school meals. Sections of the Liberal Party believed that by introducing welfare reforms, e.g. school meals, they could stave off the growth of the Labour Party which first came into Parliament early in the century. In fact, the local authority school meals system only creaked into a limited existence in the First World War, primarily to get women into the factories. Shut back after 1919, the meals service only finally boomed in the Second World War.

After the First World War, institutions which had been put into place to control food policy and to provide enough food for a beleaguered nation were rolled back. As Lord Runciman put it, it was to be 'business as usual'. The UK's first Ministry of Food was closed. State intervention in food policy, other than for trade and the occasional welfare reform, was deemed beyond the pale. Small wonder then that in the 1920s and 1930s hunger became the great issue. It is also no accident that the historian of the first Ministry of Food, William (later Lord) Beveridge was both the historian and senior civil servant of the First World War Ministry of Food. His vision of food policy was that sensible state welfare safety nets could, except in emergency times of war, obviate the need for food policy intervention.[18]

The Second World War and its Ministry of Food was the UK's one great modern experiment at a progressive, humanitarian, interventionist food policy. I don't want to go into the history of that experiment, except to say that in many respects it provided the first counter-weight to a trade-led food policy.[19] A wider range of food-related disciplines were drawn upon to inform the Ministry of Food. They worked out the dietary needs of different social groups. They prioritised policy measures on the basis of equity. The need to provide food for *all* was a paramount policy aim.

The post-war food revolution

After the Second World War, UK agricultural and food scientists and companies did what they were asked to do. The 1947 Agriculture Act, ushered in by the Labour Minister of Agriculture, Tom Williams, encouraged primary food industries to produce, produce, produce. They did so.

The food revolution of the post-war period began. What departed at the same time was any notion of a food policy as a coordination of diverse strands. A safe food policy has to include not only agriculture policy, but also health, trade, education, research and social policy. The notion of balancing production and consumption in its broadest sense died before the new goddess of production.

Symbolically, in the mid-1950s the Ministry of Food was wound up and merged into the Ministry of Agriculture and Fisheries, to give the hybrid we have today where food comes symbolically last: the Ministry of Agriculture, Fisheries and Food.

Ironically just when food policy, as distinct from agricultural policy, was demoted as a public strategy, a food revolution giving primacy and priority to production broke out. The era of intensification – from farm to factory to shop to kitchen – was ushered in.

New foods, processes, products, styles, means of cooking, handling and packaging foods came on stream. Literally thousands of new products, evidence of the fabulous creativity and imagination of food scientists and technologists, were created by millions of employees. Food manufacturing and retailing were huge employers. In the 1980s, with the collapse of the UK manufacturing base and the rise of the so-called 'service economy', catering became the huge employer (see Table I).

Table I: The food industry is a major employer
(one in seven of all workers works with food)

Sector	Numbers employed (thousands)		% females
	1981 *	1982 †	1988
Agriculture, forestry and fishing	354.6	322.0	na
Food, drink and tobacco manufacturing	658.9	548.7	42
Distribution and retail: wholesale	251.2	259.9	35
retail	572.0	624.2	64
Hotel and catering ‡	900.7	1148.9	66
Total in waged employment	2,737.4	2,903.7	

Notes: *December 1981 figures; † December 1988 figures; ‡ includes restaurants, snack bars, cafes, pubs, canteens, hotels and so on, but not public service catering.
Source: Department of Environment Gazettes.

The post-war food revolution has been marked by the new agricultural techniques, which allowed a rapid decline in employment on the land. As the table shows, there is now a significant food labour force off the land. Indeed the changing balances of power between the different sectors of the food economy – agriculture, agricultural inputs, food manufacturing, retailing, distribution, catering and consumption – is one of the most interesting things to observe about post-war British food history.

By the end of the 1980s, with a little help from the price war ushered in by the ending of Retail Price Maintenance, the food economy was dominated by retailers. They mediated between production and consumption. They were also highly concentrated.

British food manufacturers, dependent upon the retailers, concentrated dramatically, both within food sectors and by internationalisation. In most processed food products, one or two companies will dwarf others in size. This applies whether we look at bread, sausages, biscuits, drinks or confectionery. In bread for instance, two companies have around two-thirds of the UK market.

By the late 1980s these very powerful food manufacturers had already internationalised, whereas retailers had only just begun to do so. Table II indicates how successful UK food manufacturing capital was in this process. It shows that Britain had 15 of Europe's top 25 food manufacturers, by market capitalization.

Let us be clear. The post-war food revolution has brought many advantages to the ordinary member of the public. More choice, a better range of foods and availability of exciting cultural diversity. Potentially gone are the days of the parody of a boring British sludge diet! A decline in the percentage of the household's expenditure going on food is often trumpeted as evidence of economic progress. Not all agree on this, and certainly nutritionists are unhappy that there is a defeat in the sense that food-related causes are numbers one and two in the league of causes of death: CHD and cancers.[20,21]

The smaller the percentage of the household expenditure going on food means more expenditure can be spent on other household goods. The counter-argument to this is somewhat elitist in that it argues that the cheap food policy in place since the free traders won the argument over the agricultural protectionists a century ago, has allowed the British mass population to undervalue its food. I personally think this latter argument is over-simple and can lend itself to blaming the people for their own downfall. Blaming the victim makes for as poor social history as it does public health!

That said, there are problems with British food culture – but not just to do with price. Cheap food was sold to the British as one of the advantages of having colonies. Rural life was synonymous with what Marx in a memorable and arrogant phrase called the 'idiocy of rural life'. Even in the nineteenth century working people were aware that the quality of food was as important as the price and that cheap food was only an opportunity to lower wages. These realisations gave birth to the Cooperative movement.[22]

Table II: Major European food manufacturers

Company	Activity	Nationality	Market capitalization approx (£bn)
Unilever	Foods, detergents, chemicals	UK/Netherlands	8.5
Nestlé	Food manufacturing	Swiss	6.5
BSN	Food and glass products	France	2.6
Cadbury Schweppes	Manufacture of confectionery and soft drinks	UK	2.2
Associated British Foods	Food manufacturing and retail	UK	1.3
Rank Hovis McDougall	Manufacture, processing and retailing of food products	UK	1.3
United Biscuits	Manufacture and sale of food products	UK	1.2
Hillsdown	Food manufacture, furniture and property	UK	1.2
Suchard	Coffee and chocolate manufacturers	Swiss	1.1
Source Perrier	Mineral water	France	1.0
S&W Berisford	Food, financial services, property and commodities	UK	0.8
Dalgety	Agribusiness, food manufacture and commodities	UK	0.7
Unigate	Manufacture and distribution of food, transport etc.	UK	0.6
Northern Foods	Manufacture of foodstuffs	UK	0.6
Tate and Lyle	Agribusiness, sugar refining, malting, distribution, insurance	UK	0.6
Booker	Agribusiness, health products, food distribution	UK	0.6
Beghin-Say	Sugar and paper products	France	0.6

Source: *Financial Times*/CL – Alexanders Laing and Cruickshank, November 1988.

We should be wary of over-crude models of food behaviour and food culture, whether they be espoused by food and health 'missionaries' or junk-food merchants. One of the challenges which even a cursory review of the food history of one small part of the globe shows us is that we need to develop a better understanding of what moulds food behaviour and of how change occurs. This is a point not lost on those with major investments in the food economy. That is why an extremely witty and sophisticated advertising industry tickles our purses – not solely to mould our consciousness, but also to act as a barrier to would-be market entrants. Ah, the mysteries and value of brand loyalty!

In 1988 nearly half a billion pounds was spent on food advertising (see Table III). If you look at the foods advertised, they hardly deserve the title 'healthy'. I will explain why I doubt the value of cereals later, when I explore what is in breakfast cereals.

Table III: Amount spent on food advertising in 1988

	£m
Chocolate	81.7
Cereals	61.2
Coffee	55.1
Sauces, pickles, salad cream	29.2
Margarine	25.5
Tea	25.1
Frozen meals	23.6
Potato crisps and snacks	20.9
Sugar confectionery	19.6
Biscuits	19.0
Fresh and frozen poultry, meat	16.5
Meat and vegetable extracts	15.9
Milk and milk products	14.7
Cheese	14.3
Butter	9.7

Source: MEAL/Euromonitor.

The food revolution examined
I now want to explore the impact on public health, consumers and environment of the post-war food revolution. I want to analyze the 'nature, substance and quality' of some foods, to use the Food Act's phrase. I want to ask: did consumers demand what they got? I also want to reconnect the new consumer movement with the old, but first, let us explore what we mean by this phrase 'consumer'.

New consumers for old?
In the post-Second World War period, there have been three discernible phases and styles of consumer movements.

For the first post-war consumer movement, the focus was on value-for-money, information and labelling. Is this food or fridge or washing machine better value for money than that? Is the consumer being told what he or she buys? Brilliantly successful and premised upon rising consumption and the post-war Keynesian growth economics, this value-for-money thinking has been broadened and sometimes implicitly challenged by succeeding waves of consumerism.

The second wave, which I term the public interest consumer movement, was ushered in by the tough, investigative, anti-corporatist consumer work associated with Ralph Nader. Large corporations, he argued, could not be trusted to look after ordinary consumers' interest. The public interest groups' task was to champion the individual: 'us' versus 'them'.

The third wave might best be called the ecological consumer movement. Building on the experience of earlier generations, it asks about the product's quality. What of its impact, not just on the consumer's pocket but on health, the environment, distant parts of the world? What are the implications of this product, it asks? Heavily influenced by both the new public health and the environmental movements, this third wave questions the technological fetishism of post-war growth. It raises the questions of need. Why is this process or product needed? Who says so? On what grounds?

Both in my work in food policy and outside, I freely confess that I am influenced and indebted to all three consumer movement waves. What follows draws heavily on the work of the London Food Commission. I should stress that many other organisations share these perspectives. One of the joys of the late 1980s in UK food policy has been to witness the gradual coalition and bridge-building between the waves of consumer bodies. Maybe this has not a little to do with the common experience of seeing through rhetoric about consumer power.

The consumer-producer bargain collapses, as does confidence, when it emerges that consumers are not told on a packet what their food might contain, whether this hidden ingredient be fats, sugar or contaminants.

At the heart of the new food debate is the older, nineteenth-century debate which I have sketched above. Is food an individual's responsibility or a public responsibility? Is food policy a private affair or an environmental and public health matter? Can resolving problems be left to the free market or must there be protection?

To prevent food poisoning or to cure it? This became academic when the UK public found out that a staggering two-thirds of frozen chickens were found by Government scientists to be carrying salmonella.[23] Exhorting consumers to cook their chickens properly and to clean up their act flouts public hygiene principles.

Inevitably, as food policy crept up the UK public agenda in the 1980s, public reaction was unerringly appropriate. Food should be of the 'nature, quality and substance demanded'. No one goes shopping for salmonella (with some meat wrapped round it!). Attention inevitably focused on what happened to food *before* the consumer got it.

Feedstuffs

Take the feed fed to animals. In 1987, 21 out of 83 UK protein processing plants were found to be contaminated with salmonella, but there were no prosecutions. In 1988 contamination was still found – some in the same plants previously found to be contaminated. Again, there were no prosecutions.[24]

In 1988 and 1989 the public became increasingly aware of a new disease, now known as 'mad cow disease' or bovine spongiform encephalopathy (BSE). Its aetiology is not 100% clear, but is linked in all probability to feedstuffs containing sheep remains contaminated with scrapie, a spongiform disease among sheep. It is almost completely limited to the UK, and is part of a family of diseases linked to Creutzfeld-Jacob disease (CJD). In 1989 cases were running at about 400 to 500 confirmed per month. Controls were belatedly put in place, but done none the less. Feed once again was implemented. The UK is now in a *de facto* quarantine status for some aspects of animal trade.

The third feedstuff scandal concerned lead contamination of animal feedstuffs from the East, via Holland, and led to lead poisoning on 1,880 farms. The common theme that emerged from each of these feedstuff scandals was the failure of public health controls. New disease highlights the need for tight and preventive inspection. Too often, the inspection bodies are running miles behind the impact of new distribution systems and technologies.

Farms

On farms the food revolution takes its most highly publicised form: fertilisers, pesticides, the agrochemical revolution. This has all meant unnecessary residues in food, water and the environment. I won't catalogue these but merely want to pose a public health question: who gets the benefit of doubt in matters of scientific judgement? Should the benefit of doubt over new technologies and methods of producing food go, in advance of complete public health impact assessments, to production or to consumers and health? Experience shows that far too often it goes to production, not wilfully or by conspiracy, but by default. The state machine, both central and local, has been unable to exert preventive leverage; hence the public's outrage. It thought it *was* being protected.

The example of an agrochemical used on apples is a case in point. Daminozide is a cosmetic agrochemical, a plant growth regulator, which was applied to 7–10% of the British apple and pear crop prior to being withdrawn from use after a US-led scandal about possible tumour causation in 1989. In the scientific literature, there had been a trickle of papers indicating problems with daminozide from the late 1970s on. Studies done by the US environmental protection agency, the US military and others, all came to a head in 1989 when a voluntary group, the Natural Resources Defense Council of the United States, produced a large study expressing alarm at the dangers, particularly from the metabolite UDMH in processed apple products, such as apple juice.[25]

Health-conscious parents felt their good intentions undermined by a failure of public health regulation. Why, they asked, was such an unnecessary product being used without them being asked? Why weren't they told? The British

Ministry's Advisory Committee on Pesticides argued that there is no problem with daminozide. The scientific issue almost became secondary to the consumer-led question about need. Retailers imposed bans on daminozide in specifications.

Pesticides have contributed a consistent trickle of public concern throughout the 1970s and '80s. One study, done by the US National Research Council for the Environmental Protection Agency, concluded that 30% of insecticides, 60% of herbicides and 90% of fungicides could cause tumours.[26] It concluded that the 15 most risky foods from pesticides with regard to cancer in the US diet were: tomatoes, beef, potatoes, oranges, lettuce, apples, peaches, pork, wheat, soya beans, carrots, chickens, corn and grapes.

With the exception of the meat products, perhaps, these commodities are clearly acceptable components of what in the National Advisory Committee on Nutrition Education, (NACNE) and the Department of Health's Committee on Medical Aspects of Food Policy (COMA) say the public should eat more of.

To the health educators and to academics, pesticide residues on food may be a non-issue. To the consumer, they are. They weren't 'demanded'. No wonder UK farmers have been bemused by the vehemence of consumer questions in the 1980s.

Capital-intensive agriculture has clearly increased food production in terms of capacity per farm or per unit of labour. Equally, risks have been transferred and taken with too little public consultation.

Factories

The British diet is notoriously processed: 70% of the UK diet is from processed foods, according to the Cabinet Office's Advisory Committee on Agriculture Research and Development (ACARD).[27] Does this reliance on processing before the kitchen matter? Not for the first time, mixed messages emerge. On the one hand, people vote with their purses. On the other hand, there has been growing unease about what processing entails. Additives in the public mind became a symbol of the adulteration of the British diet.

The Ministry of Agriculture, Fisheries and Food's own attitude survey on additives suggested in the mid-1980s a deep public unease about the use of additives.[28] Around one-third of the sample felt all additives should be banned.

The health educators used to say that additives were a non-issue, a deviation from the big issue of heart disease and fats, salt, sugar, fibre. People like Dr Erik Millstone, Caroline Walker and Dr Melanie Miller disagreed and launched the Food Additives Campaign Team, a coalition of over 20 organisations. Additives, they argued, are what enable what the food industry calls 'non-food food' to be sold looking like real food. Many of the additives in use in the United Kingdom, and elsewhere, are purely cosmetic.[29,30] Additives disguise the food's 'nature, quality and substance'. Table IV, drawn from Mel Miller's work, reviews the main types of additives in use in the UK. The existence of 3,500 flavours in UK processed food is surely a comment on our diet.

If we take colours and compare the UK's approval system with other countries

(Table V) you will note that the UK approves many artificial colours that other countries, supposedly using high standards of food science as well, do not approve of. If you look at Norway, you'll see that they have made a policy decision to minimise or indeed ban the use of artificial colours in order to encourage the production of 'real food'. In the mid-1970s Norway took a state decision to integrate its food, agriculture, health and industry policy.

Table VI gives more examples of the role of colour in making non-food foods look like real foods; this time it is fruit drinks.

The food revolution in the factory has not just been an issue of additives. Table VII gives the total fat, sugar and salt content of British biscuits – a food the British eat an awful lot of. Without full nutrition labelling, such ingredients remain hidden from consumers' eyes.

Table IV: Main types of additives

		Approximate no.
Cosmetic additives:		3,640+
Colours	50	
Flavours	3,500+	
Flavour enhancers	7	
Sweeteners	13	
Texture modifiers	70	
Preservatives		63
Preservatives	43	
Antioxidants	13	
Sequesterants	7	
Processing aids		91
Total additives		3,794+

Source: London Food Commission: *Food Adulteration and How to Beat It,* Unwin Hyman, 1988.

Health educators are often wary, nay weary, of being seen as kill-joys. Let me come clean. I love an ice cream now and again. Table VIII reviews some well-known brands, and shows why if I have an ice cream I like it to be either a soya-based low fat substitute or else the whole full fat hog!

Take the amount of sugar in baby juice drinks. Table IX allows the consumer to ask: is it really good public health, let alone food policy, to sell well-known brand names of baby juice drinks which amount to two, three or four tea-spoonsful of sugar in a 125 ml bottle?

Table X gives the amount of sugar in fruit juices and drinks. Translated into the equivalent of sugar lumps, you will find that the British public is being sold something that sounds healthy but contains wholly unnecessary added sugar. And look at the major-selling brands of sparkling drinks. No comment.

Table XI looks at the amount of sugar in baby rusks. The message comes over with monotonous consistency. Our children's diets are starting off in what we may politely call a less than wholesome and appropriate way. Table XII gives the sugar content of leading breakfast cereals comparing them with some fairly common UK sweets. You will note that the products aimed at young children are marked for their high sugar content.

The most exasperated parent will tell you that it's better to put sugar on a cereal and get the child to eat it, than to see the child starve. This is a vicious circle, however sympathetic we may be or however we may identify from experience.

The 'sweet tooth' food culture poses a challenge both to food manufacturing and to parents, health education and public health policy. The advertising expenditure on these products indicates the need of a powerful food manufacturing sector to reinforce brands. The value of brands now features in corporate assessments of their own worth – particularly in take-over time.

Breakfast cereal manufacturers even manage to sell well-known brand names with unnecessarily high sodium contents (see Table XIII).

Table V: International status of UK-approved artificial colours, 1986

Colour	UK	Austria	Belgium	Denmark	Eire	France	Greece	Italy	Netherlands	Norway	Spain	Sweden	Switzerland	W. Germany	USA	Japan	Canada	Finland
E102 tartrazine	•									•								•
E104 quinoline yellow										•					•	•	•	
E107 yellow 2G	•	•	•			•	•	•	•	•	•	•	•	•	•	•	•	•
E110 sunset yellow										•	•							•
E122 carmoisine	•									•					•	•	•	•
E123 amaranth	•									•							•	
E124 ponceau 4R										•					•		•	
E127 erythrosine										•								
128 red 2G	•	•	•			•	•	•	•	•	•	•	•	•	•	•	•	•
E131 patent blue V										•					•	•	•	
E132 indigo carmine										•								
133 brilliant blue		•	•			•	•											
E142 green S										•	•				•	•	•	•
E151 black PN										•					•	•	•	•
154 brown FK		•	•	•		•	•	•	•	•	•	•	•	•	•	•	•	•
155 brown HT		•	•	•		•	•	•		•	•	•	•	•	•	•	•	•
129 allura red	•	•	•	•	•	•	•	•	•	•	•	•	?	•	•		•	•
No. additional artificial colours	0	0	0	0	0	0				0	0		1		0	1	4	2
Total no. artificial colours	16	8	11	12	16	11				13	0		10		11	7	11	9

• Indicates colour prohibited in food.

Source: London Food Commission 1986.

Table VI: Fruit and colouring in fruit drinks

	Estimated % of fruit	Price per litre ready to drink	Added colour
Britvic 55	55	£1.08	no
Capri-sun (various)	10	0.86p	no
Co-op Sun-up Tropical	under 45	0.76p	no
Del Monte Island Blend	under 55	0.53p	yes
Del Monte Orange Burst	under 45	0.53p	no
Five Alive Mixed Citrus	under 55	0.59p	no
Five Alive Tropical	under 55	0.59p	no
Libby's Orange 'C'	15	0.45p	yes
Libby's Blackcurrant 'C'	5	0.47p	yes
Libby's Hi-Juice Um Bongo	25	£1.00	no
Libby's Moon Shine	under 45	£1.00	yes
Presto Apple with Vitamin C	10	0.36p	no
Ribena Blackcurrant	5	0.59p	yes
Ribena Orange and Apricot	under 10	£1.00	no
Safeway Orange 'C'	under 45	0.47p	yes
Sainsbury's Hi-Juice Orange	15	0.80p	no
Sainsbury's Fruit Cocktail	under 45	0.79p	yes
Sainsbury's Tropical Fruit	under 45	0.55p	no
St Clements Original Orange	10	0.57p	no
St Clements Tropical Fruit	10	0.57p	no
St Michael Sunfruit	under 45	0.85p	yes
Sungold Mango Nectar	50	0.85p	no
Supreme Hi-Juice Orange	20	0.47p	no
Supreme Apple Drink	under 8	0.41p	no
Supreme Grapefruit Drink	under 45	0.41p	yes
Supreme Tropical Cocktail	under 45	0.52p	yes
Thomas Hi-Juice Orange	under 16	0.96p	no

Source: Safe Food Handbook, Ebury, London, 1990.

'What diet?' means 'what production?'

The point I'm making here is a very simple one. That the diet of the British, and indeed the diets of most industrialised populations, has to be looked at not just in terms of its apparent intake of foods, but also in the nature of the production that has given or provided those foods. To put it a different way, we need to be concerned not just about what diet people eat, but how that diet is produced, processed, marketed and sold. If people are to take responsibility for and control over their food, they need to know more about what happens before they eat the food.

Apply first-wave consumer value-for-money criteria to the methods of food production analysis and we start coming up with some more interesting approaches. Meat illustrates the differences between methods of production. The work of Professor Michael Crawford at the Institute of Zoology, Regents Park Zoo, London, has shown us how the fat content of the free-ranged warthog – country cousin of the pig – in its natural habitat in Africa can be as low as 1–2%, whereas the fat content of a pig may be 38–46%.[31,32] Table XIV compares different meats in a more consumer-friendly way.

Lest anyone think that I'm merely making this point at the expense of processed food from factories, look at Table XV and see the amount of added sugar given in milkshakes. Another London Food Commission colleague, Dr Tim Lobstein, in his excellent book, *Fast Food Facts*, gives you more of such information.[33] Is it really acceptable in a civilised food culture to have the equivalent of 17 lumps of sugar being added to a milk shake?

Table VII: What biscuits contain

	Total fat (g)	Per 100 g (approx. 4oz) Total sugars (g)	Sodium/salt (mg)
Sweet			
Chocolate biscuits, fully coated	28	43	160
Chocolate digestives	24	29	450
Cream sandwich (custard etc.)	26	30	220
Ginger nuts	15	36	330
Jaffa cakes	11	57	130
Plain digestives	21	14	600
Semi-sweet (Osborne, Rich Tea, Marie)	17	22	410
Short sweet (shortcake, Lincoln)	23	24	360
Shortbread	26	17	230
Wafer filled (assorted)	30	46	70
Plain			
Matzos	2	4	17
Oatcakes	18	3	1230
Rye crispbread	2	3	220
Water biscuits	13	2	470
Wholemeal crackers	11	2	700

Source: *Safe Food Handbook*, Edbury, London, 1990.

Table VIII: Value for money (ice cream)

	Additives	Double cream	Egg	Value for money
Sainsbury's	5	no	no	★★★
Loseley Dairy	2	21%	yes	★★★
Sainsbury's Dairy	4	no	yes	★★
Bejam	3	no	no	★★
Marks and Spencer	4	no	no	★
Tesco Dairy	5	1–2%	no	★
Wall's	6	no	no	★
Tesco	5	no	no	★
Iceland	5	no	no	★
Treats	6	no	no	★
Lyons Maid	5	no	no	★

Value for money is based on quality and air and water content – three stars is tops.

Source: *Safe Food Handbook*, Edbury, London, 1990.

Table IX: Sugar in baby juice drinks

	Teaspoons of sugar in 125ml (half a baby bottle), diluted as recommended
Robinson's Apple/Cherry	4.1
Robinson's Apple/Plum/Orange	4.1
Cow and Gate Pear/Peach	3.9
Cow and Gate Apple/Blackcurrant	3.5
Robinson's Apple/Orange	3.3
Delrosa Apple/Cherry	2.4
Delrosa Apple/Blackcurrant	2.4
Delrosa Apple/Orange	2.3
Cow and Gate Summer Fruits	2.2
Beecham's Baby Ribena Orange	2.0
Beecham's Baby Ribena	1.9
Robinson's Apple/Blackcurrant	1.5

Source: *Safe Food Handbook*, Edbury, London, 1990

Shops and catering

The new food revolution has occurred also in the retailing and catering sectors. The one that I've been most involved in exploring has been the cook-chill system. My colleague Julie Sheppard wrote the first independent consumer report in the United Kingdom on this method of producing 'convenience' meals.[34] 'Cook-chill' is when food is prepared, blast chilled, and kept at a low temperature, ranging from 0°C to 10°C for up to 5 days before being 'regenerated' or reheated. It's cheaper than freezing, and can give the consumer a wider range of ready-to-eat meals than via freezing. In her report, Julie Sheppard summarised a situation which can be found elsewhere in the food system.

Cook-chill technology had been introduced with too little concern for instituting proper management systems, training, cost, budgeting and auditing. To many people the most important deficiency is a failure to assess the nutrition and health impact of cook-chill food. The fact that the Department of Health approved this system of catering in 1980 without giving sufficient attention to the latter is cause for considerable concern. In particular this has become more than a concern, a scandal, due to the evidence of contamination of chilled foods by listeria.

Table X: Sugar in fruit juices and drinks

	Equivalent of sugar lumps in a 250 ml serving
Juices	
Orange juice	10
Apple juice	11
Grapefruit juice	9
Grape juice	14
Pineapple juice	11
Juice drinks	
Five Alive fruit drinks	10–12
Del Monte Island Blend drink	10
Libby's Orange 'C' drink	9
Still drinks	
Robinson's High Juice Crush	11
St Clements orange drink	11
Ribena blackcurrant drink	15
	Equivalent of sugar lumps in a 330ml can
Sparkling drinks	
Coca-Cola	13
Sparkling Ribena	16
Tizer	12
Lilt	15
Tango orange	13
7-up lemon and lime	12

Source: *Safe Food Handbook*, Ebury, London, 1990.

Table XI: Sugar in rusks

	% of added sugar in each biscuit	Cost per ounce (p)
Farley Original	31	9–15
Farex Fingers	28	8
Boots regular	26	7
Farley Low	23.5	9–15
Milupa Fruit Rusks	19.5	15
Boots Apricot Low	19	8
Cow and Gate Liga	16	12
Chocolate digestive	29	7
Ring doughnut	15	5
Plain digestive	14	4
Bread	2	3
Bikkipegs	0	41

Source: *Safe Food Handbook*, Ebury, London, 1990.

Table XII: Sugar content of breakfast cereals

	Sugars as % of weight
Bounty bar	54
Fruit gums	43
Products aimed at young children	
Sugar Puffs	57
Frosties	42
Ricicles	40
Honey Smacks	39
Coco Pops	38
Start	32
Other brand leaders	
Rice Crispies	11
Cornflakes	7
Weetabix	6
Shredded Wheat	1
Puffed Wheat	0
Products with a health image	
Sultana Bran	33
Fruit'n Fibre	27
Bran Buds	26
Country Store	24
Farmhouse Bran	23
Tropical Fruit Alpen	22
Specal K	18

Harvest Crunch	18
All Bran	15
Ready Brek (flavoured)	9
Ready Brek (unflavoured)	2
Porridge oats (quick-cook)	1
Porridge oatmeal	0

Source: Safe Food Handbook, Ebury, London, 1990.

I think we must recognise that the new technologies can create opportunities for pre-existing and 'natural' bugs such as listeria to grow. Evidence about listeria contamination in chilled foods grew following the publication of our report. The issue again was that there was insufficient control, in particular poor temperature control and knowledge. The public were *de facto* guinea pigs. In 1988 there were 287 listeriosis cases, with 61 following deaths; not a lot compared with CHD or death due to car accidents, but avoidable, and an unnecessary concern for pregnant women or people in an immuno-compromised state. No advice was given direct to pregnant women.

Retailing, precisely because it is the closest to the consumer of all the food economy sectors, has to be sensitive and quick to respond to changes in consumer market patterns. Retailers as a block have therefore been quickest to respond to the new public health, environmental and ecological consumer perspective. As Friends of the Earth have pointed out, there can often be more than a touch of green hyperbole, which is why they have launched a Green Con annual award.

The selling of products as 'environment friendly', or even ozone repairing or friendly' is a new development. In nutritional terms, the equivalent of these hypes are the contentious nutritional claims, such as foods with a band across the packet saying 'no artificial additives', but containing considerable amounts of added sugar. This is in any terms health fraud.

Table XIII: Salt content of breakfast cereals

	Sodium in a 35g serving (mg)
Highest	
Bran Flakes	300
All Bran	490
Rice Krispies	420
Special K	380
Cornflakes	370
Lowest	
Porridge oatmeal	10
Ready Brek	8
Sugar Puffs	3
Porridge oats (quick-cook)	3

Shredded Wheat	3
Puffed Wheat	1
Potato crisps, ready salted	190

Source: Safe Food Handbook, Ebury, London, 1990.

Table XIV: Meat: nutritional values and drawbacks

	Calories in 100g	Protein as % of calories	Fat as % of calories	Starch as % of calories	Good news	Warnings
Carcass meat (beef, lamb, pork)						
Joint	300	25	75	–		contaminants: fatty
Organic joint	300	25	75	–	free of contaminants	fatty
Lean meant	200	50	50	–		still fatty
Meat products (sausages, burgers, pies etc.)						
Burgers	300	33	55	12		fatty
Sausages	350	10	78	12		additives; fatty
Pies	400	10	70	20		avoid!
Poultry (chicken, turkey)						
Whole bird	250	35	65	–		
Lean meat	175	65	35	–	leaner than carcass meat	
Game (deer, rabbit, wildfowl)						
Animal	150	75	25	–	essential fats	
Bird	200	60	40	–	essential fats	

Notes: This is a rough guide only: all values are off the bone and vary considerably from joint to joint and animal to animal.

Source: Safe Food Handbook, Ebury, London, 1990.

Table XV: Added sugar in milk shakes

	Total sugars as sugars lumps
Wimpy shake (standard 400 ml)	17
McDonald's strawberry shake (regular 285 ml)	13
Average of 21 take-aways (300ml)	15
Home-made from milk shake powder (300ml)	13

Source: Safe Food Handbook, Ebury, London, 1990.

Tension points

At the end of the 1980s much has been learned and relearned about food science and food policy. But what of the future?

I want to sketch some tension points and trends I see ahead.

Europe

The first trend which will affect our food and its context is the onward march of Europeanisation. The theory about 1992, and the removal of barriers to trade by the end of that year, is this. There will be no European compositional standards. The comedians' jokes about a Euro sausage will be in the history books, not on our plates. Controls and inspections of food, notably regarding hygiene, will be at source.

There will be no inspections between point of production and point of sale. Anything sold in one member state will be deemed to be sellable in all 11 others of the European community, unless there are grounds for public health concern. In principle, there is supposed to be more information given to consumers. But what is the reality?

Public information

The track record on labelling so far has been awful – persistent delay and foot dragging by the food industry or by the British state machine. I care little which takes the major share of the blame. For decades the Committee on Medical Aspects of food policy has tacitly and sometimes overtly recommended more information to consumers. And yet at the end of the 1980s there is still a mess: labelling diversity overall, the best nutritional labelling only on own-label products (i.e. not brand names), a failure to provide codes and guidelines.

The European Community will impose some order on nutrition labels, after much horse-trading in the early 1990s. This is to be welcomed, but information and labelling doesn't just apply to nutritional issues. Many consumers want to know about pesticide residues. And here the European Community, at time of writing, is favourable only to providing a label indicating that a food has received 'post-harvest treatment'. Yet by far the most pesticide application occurs pre-harvest.

Other consumer interests also argue for information about welfare or use of biotechnology. Now the food industry argues that this will leave little room for their brand names on packets! One can have some sympathy, but they can't have it both ways. Either the consumer is to get what they demand or not. Which way are they going to jump?

Standards

Another key issue for food policy in the future will be standards. Are they going to harmonise up or down? Consumer advocates and food policy analysts unite in fearing the arrival of the lowest common denominator. This is with some justification. Table XVI gives the findings by Shropshire Trading Standards Department in the mid 1980s reviewing the meat content of processed meat products, pre and post the removal of meat product regulations in 1986.

Note that on average for over 22 products containing meat that they reviewed the minimum meat content required under the old standard was 46%. The new minimum content which they found declared on the label, after the standard was abolished, had dropped well below that to 31%. Is the consumer or the public health benefiting from this? I doubt it very much. It's not just the decline of meat (with accompanying fat content of course) that concerns me, it's what went in to replace that absent meat. And look who benefits from the removal of standards.

Table XVI: Meat content

Meat product	Minimum required meat content under old standard	New minimum meat content declared on label after standard abolished
	(%)	(%)
Roast chicken and gravy	75	45
Braised kidneys in gravy	75	70
Irish stew		
Brand A	35	25
Brand B	35	15
Minced beef with onion and gravy	50	47
Minced beef and onion	50	36
Average of 22 products	46	31

Source: Shropshire Trading Standards, 1986.

In one of the largest economic studies ever done for the European Community in pursuit of the removal of barriers to trade by the end of 1992 Paolo Cecchini produced a wonderful set of findings (see Table XVII). Please note the health-worthiness of the products for which he proclaimed the estimated cost savings to industry. The abolition of a standard for chocolate will benefit the industry by 30%! No health audit was undertaken, of course.

The European diet and market

Another trend to monitor and to attempt to influence is the shape of the European diet overall. At the time when the nutritional consensus favours the diet of the southern Europeans: low in meat, high in cereals, fresh fruit and vegetables, with fish, etc., will this diet be undermined by the invasion from the north of the over-processed, over-fatty, over-sugary diet? Remembering Professor Ancel Kays's classic study of seven countries which showed that Crete had the most wholesome diet, will the Greek diet be overtaken by the British, rather than the British by the Cretan? As someone who spends many a holiday in Greece I have more than a little interest here. Tourism has brought meat imports and raised dairy fat consumption in Greece.

Another trend to watch is market concentration. Table XVIII gives the market share of the UK grocery market for 1987–88. By the late 1980s roughly six companies dominate 70% of the UK market. Britain is not alone in this concentration. Table XIX indicates a north-south European split. Does this matter? Is this just a problem for stockbrokers? The answer is no.

The concentration of food retailing has meant a decline in the number of shops. Table **XX** gives an indication of the number of shops per thousand people. This isn't just an issue of pleasure or sociability – what could be more social than a market? – it is also an issue of availability and access. This will be writ large across Europe.

Table XVII: Cost savings from abolishing standards

Abolition of standard for traditional food	Country affected by abolition	Estimated cost saving to industry (%)
Chocolate Allowed to be made with vegetable fat instead of milk	All EC countries except Britain, Denmark and Ireland	30
Beer Allowed to contain additives and non-traditional ingredients	Germany and Greece	22
Ice cream Allowed to be made with vegetable fat instead of cream	France, Germany, Greece and Luxembourg	12
Pasta Allowed to be made with soft wheat instead of durum wheat	France, Italy and Greece	9

Abolishing traditional quality standards will reduce the cost to manufacturers of producing foods like chocolate, ice cream beer and pasta. Experience has shown that it is unlikely that these savings will be passed on to the customer.

Source: Paolo Checchini, *The European Challenge 1992*, Ec report/Wildwood House, 1988.

Table XVIII: UK grocers' market shares 1987/88

Company	Market share (%)
Tesco	14.0
J. Sainsbury	13.9
Dee (Gateway/Fine Fare)	11.5
Argyll (Presto/Safeway)	10.7
Asda	7.6
Co-op	12.1
Total	69.8

Source: Verdict Research/*Financial Times*/*Food Magazine*, spring 1989, p.19.

Table XIX: Concentration in European food retailing

	(%) of food sales 1986	
	Top 5 retailers	Top 10 retailers
Germany	60	81
Netherlands	56	79
UK	53	66
Belgium	51	66
Ireland	49	51
France	39	62
Italy	22	35
Spain	19	26
Portugal	13	15

Source: KPMG, 1989.

Table XX: Food shops per 1,000 people: Europe – north and south

Portugal	4.4
Spain	3.1
Italy	2.7
France	1.3
Germany	1.2
UK	1.0

Source: KPMG, 1989.

The issue that brings me most disquiet about immediate food policy is the question of low income and food.

Food and low income
The diet that a person eats is affected heavily by the amount of money that s/he has. Table XXI gives figures on how low-income and high-income households divide.

Table XXI: People with low incomes spend less money but a higher proportion of their income on food

	1986	
	Food expenditure per week (£)	(%) of total expenditure
Low-income households	35.84	22
High-income households	63.36	14

Source: Family Expenditure Survey 1986, HMSO, 1988.

People with low incomes spend less money but a higher proportion of their income on food. Isobel Cole-Hamilton, my colleague at the London Food Commission, has shown how in the mid 1980s the price of foods that health educators and the government itself were encouraging rose more steeply than those for less recommended foods (Table XXII).

Table XXII: In the mid-1980s the price of foods encouraged in a health diet rose more than for other, less recommended foods

	Price rise (%) 1982–86
Fish*	37
Fresh fruit*	32
Fresh vegetables*	31
Poultry*	26
Biscuits and cakes	23
Vegetable oils*	20
Bread – wholemeal	19
Whole milk	17
Bread – white	15
Meat products	14
Sugar	13
Butter	9

*Indicates foods recommended in a healthy diet.

Source: National Food Surveys 1982 and 1986, HMSO, 1984 and 1987.

What is the point of telling low-income consumers or indeed middle-income consumers to eat more fish if its price rises disproportionately more than that of other food commodities? The cost of food has to be accounted for if any sane food policy is going to be a relatively high-food-priced policy. The Second World War Ministry of Food grasped this point. Why has it been forgotten ever since?

Daily, people at the bottom of the UK social heap perform food miracles. Pound for pound people on low incomes buy nutrients more efficiently than people on higher incomes, with the exception of Vitamin C.[35] For people on low incomes price is a major, if not the major determinant of purchase patterns. Table XXIII, based upon the National Food Survey, shows that calories from fat are cheaper than those from other foods. Table XXIV shows how foods high in saturated fat tend to be cheaper than those low in fat. This study was done in a working class, multicultural area of London: Brixton.

Table XXIII: Calories from fat are cheaper than those from other foods (1986 prices)

Food	Cost of portion giving 1,000 kcal (£)
Lard and other cooking fats	0.11
Potatoes	0.22
Pasta – white	0.22
– brown	0.23
Bread – white	0.26
– wholemeal	0.37
Apples	1.61
Carrots	1.71
Oranges	1.99
Bananas	2.05

Source: National Food Survey 1986, HMSO, 1987.

Table XXIV: Foods high in saturated fat tend to be cheaper than those LOW IN FAT (December 1988 prices, Tesco, Brixton)

	Price per 1b (£)	Saturated fat per 100g (g)
Beef products:		
lean beef	2.39	2.1
fatty mince	1.20	7.3
beef sausages	0.72	10.8
Pork products:		
lean pork	2.08	3.0
fatty pork belly	0.99	15.1
pork luncheon meat	0.64	10.9
Margarines:		
polyunsaturated margarine	0.41	20.0
soft margarine	0.34	25.0
hard margarine	0.30	30.0

Source: London Food Commission

In a study done in a relatively affluent area of London, Hampstead, Cathy Mooney, the district dietitian, produced some extraordinarily simple results.[36] Table XXV shows how the cost of a 'healthy' basket of foods compared with the cost of a 'less healthy' basket of foods could be as much as 73% across a week. The baskets she compared were like for like: a full-fat cheese for a low-fat cheese, a wholemeal bread for a white sliced bread, and so on.

Table XXV: Weekly food costs

	'Healthy' basket A (£)	'Unhealthy' basket B (£)	Extra cost of basket A (%)
Deprived areas	13.84	8.02	73
Affluent areas	14.19	8.71	63

Source: Hampstead District Health Authority.

The result of studies such as these is that there is more recognition at the end of the 1980s that there is little point in telling people what is good for their health if they cannot follow that advice. Health missionaries can have little effect. If social divisions develop, rather than heal, food and health policy will have to be both sensitive and realistic.

New technologies

Ahead lies a new generation of food technologies, particularly the products of genetic engineering. A test case is in bovine sonatotropin (BST), an engineered hormone injected into cows which can increase milk yields by up to 20%. Do we really want more milk? BST is a management tool, designed for the era of milk quotas. Milk quotas – a system of control of production whereby a farmer is given a target which they cannot exceed without fine – have now become commodities in themselves. Milk quotas are bought and sold on the market by farmers. This economic lunacy will be enshrined if we allow technologies such as BST.

I am not against genetic engineering, and am at one with the Royal Commission on Environmental Pollution in saying that we must have fuller public discussion about biotechnology.[37] I regret that companies who have invested in BST have been allowed to limit public access to information, backed by the law. The Medicines Act 1968 expressly forbids the Ministry of Agriculture, Fisheries and Food from releasing the data given to it by the BST companies seeking a licence. This does little for consumer confidence, and less for scientific integrity. What is science if there can be no peer review?

Another technical development to watch will be the technical fix solution to the fat problem – fat substitutes. Table XXVI lists the companies which are developing different sorts of fat substitute. This strategy is a bit like developing sweeteners as alternatives to sugars. The new consumer approach is to ask whether they are needed in the first place. Why substitute for worthless calories? Dealing with the problem at source – in this case education – might be better for public health than substitutes.

The same moral applies to food poisoning, which continues to grow and will not be helped by removal of barriers to trade within Europe and world-wide. Health inspections, to free marketeers, are deemed hidden protectionism. In the London Food Commission's work on food irradiation, led by Tony Webb, we have concluded that there is a choice. Either the food industry and society invest in better prevention of food hygiene problems, through training, inspection, standards, etc., or they will be tempted to use irradiation which is an inadequate technical fix, at best.[38]

Irradiation damages vitamins. The proponents of irradiation say that the British suffer from a surfeit of vitamins anyway, but where is a study on the impact of the irradiation on a vegetarian diet? Our point is that irradiation is a gross irrelevancy. It is simply not needed. There are better, more sustainable ways of dealing with food poisoning. In principle, until the doubts about irradiation's safety have been resolved by independent, referenced review then the benefit of doubt over this unnecessary technology should go to the consumer.

Table XXVI: Fat substitutes

Company	Fat substitute
Arco Chemical Co (USA)	Esterified propoxylated glycerol
CPC International (USA)	Polycarboxlic acids
Ethyl Corporation (USA)	(Patent unknown)
Frito-Lay (USA)	Synthetic oils
Mitsubishi-Kaisei Food Corp (Japan)	Sucrose polyester
NutraSweet Co	Simplesse
Pfizer Inc	Polydextrose
Procter and Gamble	Olestra
Unilever NV	Sucrose polyester

Source: *Journal of the American Oil Chemists Society*, 65 (11), November 1988.

Food democracy

In the post-war period industry has done what it was asked to do: produce, produce, produce. We now know the down-side. The 1980s have been one long tussle over the shape and direction of food policy. Relations between industry, the Ministry and public have been sour, if not cynical. This is regrettable, but understandable. Ministers have consistently given priority to production interests. Table XXVII, gathered from a parliamentary question, indicates the number of meetings the Minister held with different interest groups concerned with food. I have to say that the meeting with me as representing the London Food Commission was the only one that I ever had in five and a half years!

Table XXVII: Ministerial meetings during 1988

	Meetings
National Farmers Union	37
UK Agricultural Supply Trade Association	7
Royal Society for the Protection of Birds	4
Council for the Protection of Rural England	2
National Consumer Council	2
London Food Commission	1
Royal Society for Nature Conservation	0
World Wide Fund for Nature	0
Friends of the Earth	0
Consumers in the European Community Group	0

Source: Parliamentary Question by Dr David Clarke MP.

The structure of decision making must be modernised. The imbalance between public and industry must shift. The Food Advisory Committee, which is the key Ministry of Agriculture, Fisheries and Foods committee, was given one consumer representative by the Minister, after considerable consumer pressure. In late 1989 another was added, but the domination by food industry-related personnel is still nothing short of scandalous (Table XXVIII).

Democracy is not just a question of numbers of places, but also of the spirit and style of decision making. Take irradiation. Whenever irradiation has gone out to open discussion and consultation it has been rejected. The Consumer Consultative Committee of the European Community has turned it down, but was ignored. When the European Parliament and the Environment and Consumer Protection Committee has debated the issue it too has turned it down, but has been ignored. Are these the reactions of ill-informed neurotic consumers? Even food scientists become politicians and indeed sit on these bodies!

In a promising trial, Denmark hosted a consensus conference to review food irradiation.[39] Under the auspices of the Board of Technology, a panel heard specialists chosen to represent pro, ambivalent and anti positions. A draft report was written up, and then had to be defended back before those same specialists. Contentious issues ultimately have to be resolved, if public confidence is to be retained.

Rose-tinted spectacles about European democracy have to be put firmly to one side, however. For example, the European Community's Advisory Committee on Foodstuffs, which has consumer members, has not met in 18 months. Meanwhile an *ad hoc* European Community Working Group on additives, made up of only industry and governments, has met many times. Additive harmonisation prior to the end of 1992 is a highly sensitive issue.

Consumers and public health specialists alike need to be better educated about how decisions are made in Europe. Figure 3, in graphic form, produced by the UK Consumers' Association, indicates how a food additive goes through a decision-making process.

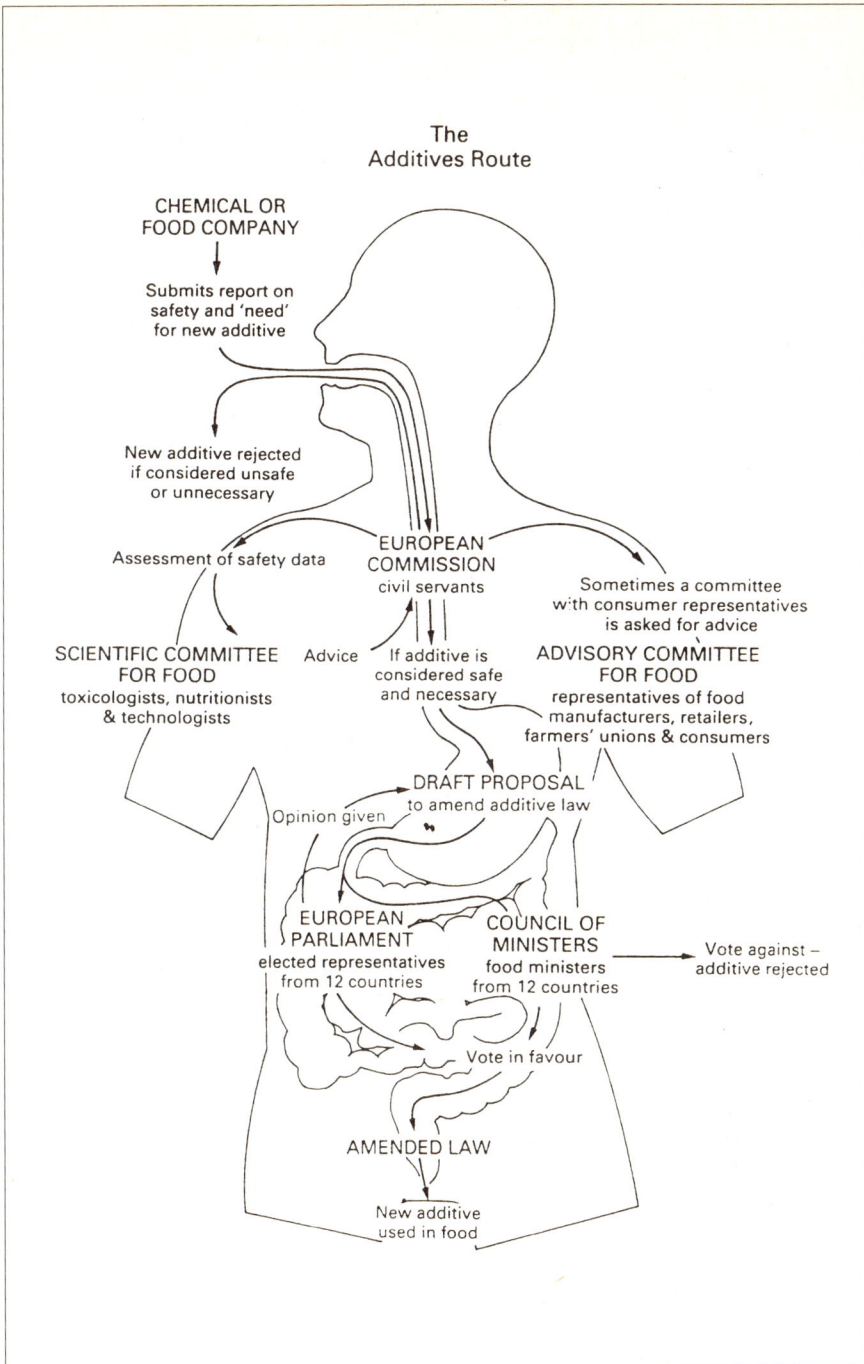

The
Additives Route

CHEMICAL OR
FOOD COMPANY

Submits report on
safety and 'need'
for new additive

New additive rejected
if considered unsafe
or unnecessary

Assessment of safety data

EUROPEAN
COMMISSION
civil servants

Sometimes a committee
with consumer representatives
is asked for advice

SCIENTIFIC COMMITTEE
FOR FOOD
toxicologists, nutritionists
& technologists

Advice

If additive is
considered safe
and necessary

ADVISORY COMMITTEE
FOR FOOD
representatives of food
manufacturers, retailers,
farmers' unions & consumers

DRAFT PROPOSAL
to amend additive law

Opinion given

EUROPEAN
PARLIAMENT
elected representatives
from 12 countries

COUNCIL OF
MINISTERS
food ministers
from 12 countries

Vote against –
additive rejected

Vote in favour

AMENDED LAW

New additive
used in food

Figure 3. The European additives route.
Source: Consumers' Association, *Which? Way to Health*, June 1989.

Table XXVIII: Food Advisory Committee

	Consumer representatives
Food-industry related	8
Academic and medical	4
Local authority	2
Consumer advocate	1

The Food Advisory Committee is MAFF's key food policy committee.
It has been criticised for its lack of consumer representation compared
with those from industry.

Source: MAFF press release/*Food Magazine*, spring 1989.

The fourth hurdle: need

The issue of need is going to become more and more important. This is often
referred to by the fairly lugubrious phrase: the fourth hurdle. Social need, and
the application of social criteria to food products, are going to become increasingly important. From some quarters this will no doubt be seen as an
infringement of rights. Critics will say that to introduce a criterion of need to
technology assessment will be a recipe for 'neurotic, whingeing consumers' (a
phrase used by one leading food industry-sponsored technologist) to delay
progress.

The food industry constantly makes decisions on social criteria, its criteria,
about food technologies. The point at issue is not that the fourth hurdle is
going to introduce a new dimension to food decision making and auditing. The
fourth hurdle merely allows more interests to be represented at an open table.

Sustainability

The fourth hurdle is needed because fundamental questions about the sustainability of current food production methods have been raised. Technologies
will increasingly have to be judged by broadened criteria of efficiency and worth.
The new wave of ecological consumers are forerunners of a deep challenge to
the food system. Can it survive on current methods of production?

Quite what will emerge as a sustainable system is unclear. To the environ-
mentally conscious consumer, packaging is waste. To the student of hygiene,
packaging is a necessary public health measure. The gap must be bridged or
sustainability will mean different things to different people.

A shopping list for the future

Before us lies a great challenge. Are we going to develop a new philosophy of
health, sustainability and welfare for land, food production, animals and ourselves? Or are we going to carry on walking down the same old road? I think
we deserve better than that. Here are some key issues that I think we must
address.

Reform of the Ministry of Agriculture, Fisheries and Food is long overdue.

I would like the Ministry to become a Ministry of Food covering the entire food economy. It needs a consumer division within it, with better coordination between government ministries and with voluntary bodies outside it.

There should be a Food Policy Coordination Committee, perhaps at Cabinet or sub-Cabinet level. An independent Food Standards and Safety Executive should be set up, perhaps modelled on the Health and Safety Executive. This should learn from the successes and failures of other agencies, such as the Food and Drug Administration in the United States.

Complete nutritional labelling, and other forms of labelling as well, are essential to any new consumer-producer pact. If consumers eat the food, they have the right to know more about it. This means – the thrust of this paper's argument – that the consumer has a right to know about how the food is produced, not just what it is.

Food policy should operate on democratic and equitable bases. To that end, there should be an annual food policy review, much as the Chief Medical Officer produces a health review. I would like to see an annual Food Policy Conference bringing together all sides of the food economy. I would also like to see an independent Consumer Food Policy Conference. In an ideal world, these could work together. Is the UK quite ready for that?

Quality standards should be set, in principle, to optimum levels. There should be controls on adulterating, bulking agents. Mechanically recovered meat (MRM), a sludge produced from the by-products of the butchery trade, is allowed into meat products up to 10% by content without declaration, despite the Food Standards Committee's declaration in 1980 that it was microbiologically less stable than carcass meat. MRM should be banned.

A new system of social impact statements should be developed by the new Ministry of Food. Social impact statements, first argued for by the Working Party on Low Income and Food by the London Food Commission,[40] are a relatively simple way of getting decision makers – civil servants and food industry alike – to think through the potential impact of products. This is not a block on progress but merely enables anticipation of problems.

Product liability laws need to be toughened up. The Consumer Protection Act currently does not apply to food. It should. Food premises should be licensed. Other countries have systems of training and licensing their food handlers. Food handlers should be inspected and examined. We apply such thinking to our automobiles and our drivers. Why not food?

There should be a public health-oriented enquiry into the role of the UK's concentrated food industries. I would like to see an inquiry by the Monopolies and Mergers Commission and the Office of Fair Trading.

We need also, last but not least, a measure, a drive on public food education. The principle of 'caveat emptor' – let the buyer beware – is no way to run a food policy. Consumers are always the last line of defence on issues such as hygiene and nutrition. They should not be the only line of defence. The sane way to progress is to ensure that excellent standards of information and education, skills and training apply throughout the food chain.

There is no reason why the future and present consuming public could not begin to have integrated education at school. Without an integrated food policy and the structures to go with it, such as a coordination committee bringing together the work of the Ministry of Agriculture, Fisheries and Food with the Department of Education and Science, there will be no progress.

I am an optimist. Major problems have come to light. They can and must be resolved.

References

1. Fenelon, K.G. (1952). *Britain's Food Supplies*. London: Methuen, Ch. 10.
2. Tracy, M. (1982). *Agriculture in Western Europe*. London: Granada.
3. Body, Sir Richard (1982). *Agriculture: the Triumph and the Shame*. London: Temple Smith.
4. Body, Sir Richard (1984). *Farming in the Clouds*. London: Temple Smith.
5. Lang, T. (1988). 1992 – trading in standards. *Food Magazine*, October, 10–11.
6. Consumers in the European Community Group (1987). *A Hot Potato? Food Policy in the EEC*. London: CECG.
7. Consumers in the European Community Group (1987). *Could do Better: Towards an EEC Policy for Consumers*. London: CECG.
8. Walker, C. & Cannon, G. (1984). *The Food Scandal*. London: Ebury.
9. Health Education Council (1983). *Report of the National Advisory Committee on Nutrition Education*. London: Health Education Council.
10. Organization for Economic Co-operation and Development (1981). *Food Policy*. Paris: OECD, Ch. 1.
11. Paulus, I. (1974). *The Search for Pure Food*. Oxford: Martin Robertson.
12. London Food Commission (1988). *Food Adulteration and How to Beat It*. London: Unwin.
13. Semmel, B. (1960). *Imperialism and Social Reform*. London: Allen and Unwin.
14. Clutterbuck, C. & Lang, T. (1982). *More Than we can Chew*, London: Pluto.
15. Burnet, J. (1968). *Plenty and Want: a Social History of Diet in England*. Harmondsworth: Penguin.
16. Lang, T. (1981). *Now You See Them, Now You Don't*. Rochdale: Rochdale Alternative Press.
17. Le Gros Clarke, F. & Titmuss, R. (1939). *Our Food Problem and its Relation to National Defenses*. Harmondsworth: Penguin.
18. Beveridge, W. (1928). *Food Control*. London: Oxford University Press.
19. Hammond, R. (1956). *Food*, Vols 1, 2 and 3. London: HMSO and Longman, Green.
20. Committee on Medical Aspects of Food Policy (COMA) – DHSS (1984). *Diet and Cardiovascular Disease*. London: HMSO.
21. World Health Organization, Regional Office for Europe (1988). *Healthy Nutrition*. Copenhagen: WHO Regional Publications European Series no. 24.
22. Redfern, P. (1913). *The Story of the CWS 1863–1913*. Manchester: Co-operative Wholesale Society.
23. London Food Commission (1988). Communicable Diseases Surveillance Centre data 1987. In: *London Food Commission on Food Adulteration*. London: Unwin-Hyman, p. 244.

24. Lang, T. (1989) *Report on Salmonella and Eggs*. Evidence submitted to the House of Commons Agriculture Select Committee, London: HMSO.

25. Natural Resources Defense Council (1989). *Intolerable Risk*. New York: NRDC.

26. National Research Council (1987). *Regulating Pesticides*. Washington, DC: National Academy Press.

27. ACARD (1982). *The Food Industry and Technology*. London: HMSO.

28. MAFF and Consumers' Association (1985). *Survey on Additives*. London: MAFF.

29. Millstone, E. (1986). *Food Additives*. Harmondsworth: Penguin.

30. Lawrence, F. (ed.) (1986). *Additives – a survival guide*. London: Century.

31. Crawford, M. & Marsh, D. (1989). *The Driving Force*. London: Heinemann.

32. Crawford, M. & Crawford, S. (1972). *What we Eat Today*. London: Spearman.

33. Lobstein, T. (1988). *Fast Food Facts*. London: Camden Press.

34. Sheppard, J. (1987). *The Big Chill*. London: London Food Commission.

35. Cole Hamilton, I. & Lang, T. (1986) *Tightening Belts*. London: London Food Commission.

36. Mooney, C. (1988). A Healthy Diet: who can afford it?, *Food Magazine*, October, 20.

37. Royal Commission on Environmental Pollution (1989). *13th Report, House of Lords*. London: HMSO.

38. Webb, T. & Lang, T. (1990). *Food Irradiation: the Myth and the Reality*, Wellingborough: Thorsons.

39. Danish Technology Board (Teknologienaevnet) (1989). Final document on Consensus Conference on Food irradiation 22nd- 24th May 1989, Copenhagen: DTB.

40. Cole Hamilton, I. & Lang, T. (1986). *Tightening Belts*. London: London Food Commission.

Childhood Cancer and Nuclear Installations

Public Health (1991), 105, 277–285. © The Society of Public Health, 1991. 8th Duncan Memorial Lecture University of Liverpool, 5th December 1990. M. J. Gardner. Professor of Medical Statistics, MRC Environmental Epidemiology Unit, (University of Southampton), Southampton General Hospital, Southampton SO9 4XY.

Introduction

Dr William Henry Duncan was the first man in the country to be given the title of Medical Officer of Health and Liverpool was the first city to have such a post. Dr Duncan was of course a remarkable man and the fact of his appointment as Medical Officer of Health was a realisation of much that he had done before that date in 1847 to consider the reasons why the health of some people living in Liverpool was less satisfactory than others.

The first Duncan Memorial Lecturer seven years ago in 1983 was the late Dr Sidney Chave and he described very adeptly in his lecture the life and activities of Dr Duncan – I would suggest that it is recommended reading for anybody who has not yet done so.[1] One of the subsequent lectures was given by Sir George Godber, a former Chief Medical Officer, and he traced the history of Medical Officers of Health from the time of Duncan onwards.[2] Another more recent Duncan Memorial Lecture was given by the present Chief Medical Officer, Sir Donald Acheson, who examined the state of public health in this country.[3] My topic is somewhat narrower than either of these but addresses a problem that has emerged in the last few years and which had been the cause of some anxiety and much activity. My plan is to try to describe the picture to you and put the current view in some perspective.

However, I thought that I would start off by staying with the time of Duncan for a short while. Soon after Dr Duncan became Medical Officer of Health for Liverpool in 1847, it became a legal requirement that each death in this country had to be registered and for the cause of death to be certified – this took place in 1850. One of the things that emerged as a consequence was the ability to look at the public health on a geographical basis around the country in a way that had not been possible before, and in the 1870s there became available maps for England and Wales showing the picture of fatal disease by area.

Cancer in the 1850s

The first maps that I know of were produced by a surgeon at St Bartholomew's

Hospital in London called Alfred Haviland and, to consider one example, he produced a map of mortality from cancer of all types in women for the years 1851–1860.[4] The general picture that he commented on was of lower cancer death rates in the west of the country with higher rates in the east. His explanations for these differences were nearly all in terms of geophysical factors. He mentioned, for example, that on the west side of the country there are elevated hilly and mountainous areas, with geologically old formations of hard rock, which are well drained by rivers flowing down to the sea. On the east side of the country, however, the landscape is different. It is low-lying, with more recent geological formations of chalk and other soft rock, where the rivers tend to flow in valleys and flood.

To quote from Haviland's text, he commented that: 'The maps teach us that the high, dry sites on the older rocks are the places where cancer does not thrive, and that it does thrive in the vales by the sides of large rivers which overflow their banks, and in the neighbourhood of which are to be found the drifts of ages of washing from the inhabited country above. When there is a tendency to cancer let the patient be removed to the high dry sites; and perchance if whole families were thus to emigrate, we should not hear so much of the hereditary character of this and many other diseases.' This paragraph is just a short abstract from a remarkable book. The point that comes over is that almost his total explanation of the geographical distribution of cancer was in relation to the geophysical environment. However, as you will have noticed, Haviland was also thinking ahead from causation to prevention, through the idea of moving people to the areas with low rates from those with high cancer mortality. Appropriately, in the context of the Duncan Lecture, Haviland was also one of the first Medical Officers of Health – for Northamptonshire, Leicestershire, Rutland and Buckinghamshire.

It is interesting to reflect that in 1875, when writing the text, Haviland remarked that he thought it worthwhile to produce a map of cancer for women, but not for men, because the number of deaths from cancer among men was far fewer than among women. During the 1850s, in fact, the number of cancer deaths among women was about three times that among men. Of course, the sex ratio has reversed since then – not to the same degree – so that cancer death rates are now higher in men than women. There are two main reasons why this change has happened. First, ever since 1850, the principal cancer in women has remained cancer of the breast. This dominated the cancers that were diagnosed during 1851–60, and is why female cancer was higher than male. Secondly, the fact that cancer death rates in men are now higher than in women is because they are dominated by cigarette-related lung cancer cases. Without these the death rates from cancer in women would still be 25% higher than in men. It is an interesting change that has taken place over a period of just over 100 years, from cancer reporting being markedly more common among women to cancer being slightly more common among men.

Cancer in the 1970s

As far as the Merseyside area goes, cancer rates in women in the 1850s were among the lowest in the country. Has the pattern changed since then? A more recent map gave cancer death rates among women during 1968–1978 by local authority areas such as county boroughs and rural districts, and showed that areas with high cancer death rates and those with low cancer death rates were spread around the country.[5] However, Merseyside had rates during the 1970s that were among the highest in the country. In particular, the overall cancer rates in Liverpool and surrounding areas were some 10–30% above the national average. Why is this? What has changed? Well, to consider specifically first cancer of the breast, rates are low in this part of the country and the high rates are, just as they were in Haviland's days, mainly in the southern and eastern parts of the country. Thus it does not seem that the geographical distribution of breast cancer has changed much at all in over 100 years' time span. In fact, the Merseyside area as a whole had a death rate from breast cancer some 10% below the national average during the 1970s. So why is overall cancer high now among local women if breast cancer is low? The answer is because of high lung cancer rates, which are concentrated very much in London and its surrounding areas but also on Merseyside and Tyneside in particular. Specifically, lung cancer rates during the 1970s among women in this area were as much as 50% above the national figure – in Liverpool itself exactly 50% above the average for England and Wales. It is, of course, well known that this area also has one of the highest lung cancer rates among men. As part of the World Health Organisation's 'Healthy Cities' project there is a major move to remedy this situation.

Cholera and disease clusters

I want to stay with historical maps for a moment and consider a map of a different kind that was partially responsible for the discovery of the cause and prevention of one of the diseases that ravaged the country during the time of Duncan. In the Soho area of London during the month of August 1854 – seven years after Dr Duncan had been installed as Medical Officer of Health for Liverpool – there was a cholera epidemic that has been described as the most terrible outbreak which ever occurred in this kingdom. An anaesthetist called Dr John Snow, who lived about half a mile from this area, had already taken an interest in why, where and which people cholera struck.[6] His suspicions quickly fell on a well in Broad Street, and were strengthened when he discovered that 'nearly all the deaths had taken place within a short distance of the pump'. He soon established that almost all the people who had died in this particular epidemic had consumed water from the same pump. As a consequence of Snow's enquiry the pump handle was removed to stop any further people drinking water from that particular source. This was one of the first important observations which led finally to proof that cholera was a water-borne disease and, among other things, led to the sanitary revolution that later followed. So this was a success story of a cluster of disease being observed, the source being identified and later leading to the elucidation of the cause and subsequent prevention of this illness.

I have discussed this bit of medical history, contemporary with Duncan's time as Liverpool's Medical Officer of Health, because the issue as to whether clusters can lead to the elucidation of new causes of disease is still one which is the subject of much discussion and debate. One does not have to listen too hard or often to hear allegations that some disease or other is being produced in the area of a source of contamination of some nature – for example, around an incinerator, a toxic waste dump, a polluted river, or, in the case of what I want to talk about now, around a nuclear installation.

Childhood leukaemia around Sellafield

There are a number of nuclear installations within the United Kingdom, including research establishments, power generating stations and waste repro-cessing centres. In particular Windscale and Calder Hall, collectively known as Sellafield, is on the west coast of Cumbria just under 100 miles to the north of Liverpool. My own involvement with this subject started towards the end of 1983 when the Yorkshire television programme called 'Windscale: the nuclear laundry' was screened. The television producer approached the management of Sellafield with a request for their cooperation in producing a documentary on the health of the radiation workforce at Sellafield, to be told that there were no definite indications of any long-term ill-health effects of radiation exposure on their workers – which was justified and in accord with both a study that had been carried out by the company itself[7,8] and also one independently.[9] However, while in the area negotiating for the programme the producer heard incidentally of some cases of childhood leukaemia near the installation, and decided to switch the thrust of his programme to describing and discussing these childhood leukaemia cases. He finally presented a programme that suggested that there was a cluster of childhood leukaemia cases in the area near Sellafield – in particular the village of Seascale, some three kilometres to the south – and alleged that these cases were linked to the discharges of radioactive liquids from the plant to the Irish Sea, which subsequently polluted the beaches, fish and seafood. The government set up an independent enquiry under the Chairmanship of Sir Douglas Black to investigate the suggestion and allegation. I was asked to be a member of this team, not because of any detailed knowledge of childhood leukaemia or radiation biology but because of the work on cancer mapping which we were then undertaking.

Is there an Excess?

A major question is: how to tackle such an allegation? Because this has become a fairly common occurrence there are now emerging quite clear guidelines for how to go about such an investigation – and a lot of these owe much to the methods of John Snow back in the 1850s. One of the first things that needs to be done is to investigate the cases that are alleged to have occurred and to confirm that they exist in medical records – either hospital or cancer registration records, or on death certificates. If the cases are not genuine and not known to the medical profession then the allegation can effectively be discounted at that stage. On the other hand, as in this instance, if the cases are shown to be genuine then the investigation needs to go further. One of the next questions needs to be 'is there an excess?', given that the cases suggested have been confirmed. In this situation the question was addressed by carrying out geographical studies of childhood cancer in districts in the neighbourhood of Sellafield and other parts of the country.

The location of Sellafield is on the coast of West Cumbria with the village of Seascale some three kilometres to the south. Sellafield is what was called the Rural District of Ennerdale and Seascale in the Rural District of Millom – in what follows I will consider some statistics for these areas.[10] Deaths from leukaemia under 25 years of age during 1968–78 in Ennerdale were very much the same as expected on the basis of the size and age distribution of its population considering the rates for leukaemia under 25 years of age during 1968–78 in Ennerdale were very much the same as expected on the basis of the size and age distribution of its population considering the rates for leukaemia in England and Wales as a whole. However, in Millom there were six deaths compared with 1.4 expected, an excess of just over four-fold.

Dr Alan Craft and his colleagues from Newcastle looked at childhood leukaemia in the 675 electoral wards of the Northern region for which they had cancer registration details in under 15-year-olds for the years 1968–1982. Among these 675 electoral wards there were 19 that were statistically considered to have raised rates. Seascale was one of these and in a direct statistical sense could be considered to have the most extreme rate of childhood leukaemia among all the 675 wards.

It is helpful to try to put the four-fold excess that was found in Millom Rural District into context by comparing it with the other 151 Rural Districts around England and Wales of similar population size. It was not, in fact, the most extreme with one other Rural District having a slightly higher excess, but the fact that it was very near the top did indicate that the rate in that area was at least somewhat unusual. As a consequence of this evidence the conclusion of the Black Inquiry was that the suggestion of the Yorkshire television programme could not be rejected. There did seem to be an excess of childhood leukaemia in this area around Sellafield although it was based on a small number of cases and seemed to be particularly focused in the village of Seascale.

Why is there an Excess?

This then leads on to the question: 'what is the suggested cause of the excess?' I have already mentioned that the Yorkshire television programme suggested that it was related to the level of radioactive discharges from Windscale. The liquid discharges from Windscale have been substantially greater than those from any other nuclear establishment in Britain, and this is also true for airborne discharges.

The next question has to be: 'is the suggestion plausible?' It is worth looking at the evidence that suggests there is a causal relationship between exposure to ionising radiation and some cancers.[11] First of all, as examples among occupationally exposed groups of workers, it is accepted that leukaemia was caused among early radiologists, that uranium miners inhaling radon gas have had up to a five-fold increase of lung cancer and that workers who painted luminous dials on watches, using paint containing radium isotopes, developed bone cancers. It is also know that leukaemia and other cancers developed among survivors of the atomic bombs that were dropped on Hiroshima and Nagasaki during the Second World War with the leukaemias following relatively soon after the bomb and the other cancers somewhat later. As well it is clear that some patients who have had X-rays or radiotherapy have subsequently developed cancers. Examples include women developing breast cancer following X-ray of the chest after they had been treated for pulmonary tuberculosis, leukaemia among patients given radiation therapy for ankylosing spondylitis, and leukaemia again among patients with cervical cancer also treated by radiotherapy. Additionally, it is now generally accepted that antenatal X-rays of the abdomen of pregnant mothers can produce about a 50% excess risk among their children of developing leukaemia after birth. This final example is clearly a relevant one in the context of the problem being discussed. So the plausibility of the excess of childhood leukaemia in Seascale being related to radiation at Sellafield cannot be totally rejected, since we know that radiation figures quite high on the list of candidates for causing cancer – leukaemia in particular.

Other Nuclear Sites

One of the next obvious questions is to ask: 'what about near other nuclear sites?' Thus it is sensible to look at childhood leukaemia and cancer around other nuclear installations in this country.[12] First, let us consider the Scottish sites for the reason that they include Dounreay, which is the only other nuclear waste reprocessing site, apart from Sellafield, in Britain. Part of the evidence produced by the Scottish group researching this problem showed that during the years 1968–1984 there were five cases of leukaemia under age 25 years within 12.5 kilometres of Dounreay compared with about 1.5 expected. Thus, as for Sellafield, there was an excess – although it was smaller if a 25-kilometre radius was used instead of 12.5 – but apparent excesses around Hunterston and Chapel Cross were much smaller. In England and Wales during 1961–1980 leukaemia registrations, again under age 25 years, were found to be somewhat higher in areas near the nuclear installations contrasted with control areas that were taken for comparison. The installation areas were higher than the control areas, apart from Sellafield, by a figure of between 10% and 20%. As a final example consider the figures for leukaemia and also other cancers in areas around Aldermaston, Burghfield and Harwell, which are nuclear installations that have specifically been looked at by a research group based in Oxford. There appears to be a 64% increase in leukaemia among under five-year-olds in a 10-kilometre radius around these installations compared with further away, and also an apparent 24% increase in other cancers within the 10-kilometre radius. Thus I think it is possible to make a general statement that there does appear to have been an excess of childhood leukaemia around nuclear installations in the UK, although apart from Sellafield and Dounreay the excess is relatively small.

Seascale Cohort Study

I would now like to discuss in further detail the next steps that can be taken in investigating such a cluster by reference to what has taken place around Sellafield. One of the further studies that was recommended by the Black report and which has now been completed was a cohort study. This was essentially a study of all the children who were born or attended schools in Seascale during 1950–1983, which at the time of study covered most of the period of operation of the Sellafield plant. Using access to local birth registers we identified just over 1,000 children who had been born in the village during these years, and with access to school registers through the local Cumbria Education Committee and headmistresses of the schools we were able to identify just over 1,500 other children who had been born since 1950 and moved into Seascale subsequently to attend one of the three schools up to 1984. It was found that cases of leukaemia had occurred only among children born in the village with none occurring in children who moved in after birth. For other cancers there was no suggestion of any excess among those born in the village. Our conclusion at this time was that there was a genuine excess of childhood leukaemia in Seascale and if there was a genuine local factor causing this excess then it appeared to operate either very early in life or before birth.[13, 14] The next step, having determined that an excess exists – and the cohort study was carried out partly because of potential deficiencies in geographical analysis – is to look at individual factors on these cases to determine whether or not any can be established that help to explain why they have occurred.

West Cumbria Case-Control Study

This can be done by a case-control study, in which cases of a disease are compared with healthy children who have not developed the illness. So we carried out such a case-control study that had very specific objectives, which were to examine whether or not the excess was related to the causal factor that I have already mentioned, that is prenatal abdominal X-ray of the mother, whether it is related to suggested risk factors for childhood leukaemia such as viral infections or social class; or whether it is related to exposure to radiation as a result of the Sellafield nuclear site either, first, through habits which potentially enhance exposure to the radioactive discharges to sea such as playing on the beach or eating fresh fish or shellfish or, secondly, whether exposure to radiation through working at the plant is relevant. To carry out this study we ascertained all the cases of leukaemia and lymphoma (both non-Hodgkin's lymphoma and Hodgkin's disease) who had been born and diagnosed in West Cumbria during the years 1950–1985 and which had occurred under 25 years of age. We then identified, from the same birth registers as where the cases had been entered, control children of the same sex and roughly the same date of birth and who had either been born in any town within the Birth Registration District or had more specifically been born in the same village or town as the case to whom they were matched.

Without going into all the details of the results of this study,[15, 16] I can say that we found similar risks for prenatal X-rays to those identified earlier, no important risks in relation to the suggested risk factors that I mentioned, and no apparent risks in relation to exposure to radiation through the discharges. However, we did find that, among the five cases of childhood leukaemia in Seascale, the four fathers whom we fully identified and obtained radiation records for had higher exposures before their child's conception than the fathers of the comparison children who were also born in Seascale. This led to the suggestion that in some way the father's exposure to radiation during his employment at Sellafield before the conception of his child may be relevant to the subsequent development of leukaemia. When we looked at the results for non-Hodgkin's lymphoma, which were based on fewer cases, the findings were not dissimilar to leukaemia whereas for Hodgkin's disease, which has never been associated with ionising radiation in the medical literature, there was no relationship to father's employment at Sellafield as a radiation worker. At this stage we feel that the perspective has changed from that of a suggested childhood leukaemia excess in Seascale which is possibly related to environmental radiation contamination, as proposed by the Yorkshire television programme, to a confirmed childhood leukaemia excess in the village which is statistically related to father's occupational radiation exposure during his work at Sellafield before the child's conception.

Lowering radiation exposures

This finding clearly needs and is receiving more attention and detail to try to understand whether it is radiation caused and if so quite how it might operate. In the meantime it is appropriate to consider, as did Haviland and Snow – and indeed Duncan – last century, the issue of what should be done if anything to lead to 'prevention'. I think that this can be taken in two steps. First, if our results are confirmed then I think we can make a general statement that there would not seem to be a major public health problem in relationship to the radiation contamination of the environment that has undoubtedly taken place. This is a minimal statement and it is not in any way meant to imply that contamination therefore is not important. Secondly, the comment can be made that the problem would seem to be one of taking preventive measures among the workforce if anywhere.

So what has happened over the years in terms of radiation exposure levels of the workers and discharges at Sellafield? Average yearly radiation doses among workers at Sellafield were at their highest during the 1950s and have decreased since then through the 1970s and 1980s. So worker exposure to radiation has been declining. Average yearly radioactive liquid discharges to the Irish Sea from Sellafield were relatively low until the early 1970s, when they peaked, and have declined during the 1980s. So again, as for worker exposure, discharges to the sea have declined and are continuing to do so.

What else can be done? As a consequence of our case-control study there has been discussion at British Nuclear Fuels about how radiation exposures of workers can be even further reduced, in particular now among those who are contemplating having children. This has resulted in dose-reduction working groups, with representatives of various sections of the workforce and management, aimed at reducing exposure throughout the plant as much as is possible without jeopardising the work environment. In addition, contour maps for each part of the plant have been and are being produced which show the dose rate of ionising radiation that applies to each area in which workers may find themselves operating. Thus there are certainly intentions to lower the exposure levels to as low as reasonably achievable within the context of appropriate working practices

Summary

So where are we now? I think the first thing to say is that there is a well-established excess around Sellafield of childhood leukaemia, although excesses around other nuclear sites are of a lower magnitude. The excess near Sellafield is strongly associated with fathers having high exposure to external whole-body penetrating radiation while working at the installation before their child's conception. But is this association pointing towards a causal mechanism? One possibility is genetic damage, but most geneticists and radiobiologists would consider that the levels of occupational exposure, even at Sellafield, are too low for this to be a plausible pathway on current knowledge. This is based to some extent on the lack of any similar effect among children born subsequently to Japanese survivors of the atomic bombs – however, the scenario is somewhat different contrasting a high short-term exposure with a lower long-term exposure. As well, some workers at Sellafield will also be exposed to radionuclides, such as plutonium, which we have not yet been able to analyze for. In addition, there are other exposures in a complex environment which may or may not be relevant. One experimental study in the laboratory using animals supports the idea that a pathway through irradiation of the parents is plausible, although this one result needs replication.[17] Other causes have been suggested for the excess childhood leukaemia levels in particular around nuclear establishments – these include population movement,[18] implicating viruses that have long been considered to be associated with childhood leukaemia, high rates in isolated communities,[19] and also selection of areas for nuclear sites that have a natural propensity to high rates.[20]

Geographical studies have now been carried out in some other countries, such as France[21] and the United States,[22] where the excesses seen around nuclear establishments in the UK have not been observed. It may be that they genuinely do not occur but it is also possible that the geographical areas used, particularly in the United States, are too large to identify any localised effect. A similar study in Canada is less negative and is currently being extended in its coverage. There are currently two other case-control studies in the United Kingdom underway and nearing completion. The first of these is around Dounreay, the other nuclear waste reprocessing site, and the other is around the Aldermaston and Burghfield installations. The results of these studies will be of interest, of course, but how much they can be considered to be reproductions of the circumstances at Sellafield is less clear. As well, there are preliminary plans to do detailed studies around a number of the oldest nuclear installations in the United States and France.

Finally, I would mention that there are advanced intentions to carry out two major studies in an attempt to take the position further. One of these is to do a follow-up study of all the children, maybe also grandchildren, of radiation workers at Sellafield both past and present – this will give a much wider coverage than the studies that we have been able to carry out thus far. Secondly, there is a proposal to look for cases of cancer among children of all registered radiation workers in the UK regardless of their place of employment. By the nature of this kind of work these studies will take three or more years to complete, but they will both be part of exploring further the linkage of the various pieces of this jigsaw.

Acknowledgement

I would like to express my appreciation at being invited to be the Duncan Memorial Lecturer for 1990.

References

1. Chave, S. (1984). Duncan of Liverpool – and some lessons for today. *Community Medicine*, 6, 61–71.
2. Godber, G. E. (1986). Medical officers of health and health services. *Community Medicine*, 8, 1–14.
3. Acheson, E. D. (1988). On the state of the public health. *Public Health*, 5, 431–438.
4. Haviland, A. (1875). *The Geographical Distribution of Heart Disease and Dropsy, Cancer in Females and Phthisis in Females in England and Wales*. London: Smith Elder & Co.
5. Gardner, M. J., Winter, P. D., Taylor, C. P. & Acheson, E. D. (1983). *Atlas of Cancer Mortality in England and Wales, 1968–1978*. Chichester: Wiley.
6. Snow, J. (1855). *On the mode of communication of cholera*. (2nd ed. reprinted 1936, with Appendix of 1856.) New York: The Commonwealth Fund.

7. Clough, E. A. (1983). The BNFL radiation-mortality study. *Journal of the Society for Radiological Protection*, 3(1), 24–27.

8. Clough, E. A. (1983). Further report on the BNFL radiation-mortality study. *Journal of the Society for Radiological Protection*, 3(3), 18–20.

9. Smith, P. G. & Douglas, A. J. (1986). Mortality of workers at the Sellafield plant of British Nuclear Fuels, *British Medical Journal*, 293, 845–854.

10. Black, D. (1984). *Investigation of the Possible Increased Incidence of Cancer in West Cumbria*. London: HMSO.

11. Boice, J. D. & Land, C. E. (1982). Ionising radiation. In: Schottenfield, D. & Fraumeni, J. F. (eds). *Cancer Epidemiology and Prevention*. Philadelphia: Saunders, 231–253.

12. Gardner, M. J. (1989). Review of reported increases of childhood cancer rates in the vicinity of nuclear installations in the UK. *Journal of the Royal Statistical Society (Series A, Statistics in Society)*, 152, 307–325.

13. Gardner, M.J., Hall, A.J., Downes, S. & Terrell, J.D. (1987). A follow-up study of children born to mothers resident in Seascale, West Cumbria (birth cohort). *British Medical Journal*, 295, 822–827.

14. Gardner, M.J., Hall, A.J., Downes, S. & Terrell, J.D. (1987). A follow-up study of children born elsewhere but attending schools in Seascale, West Cumbria (schools cohort). *British Medical Journal*, 295, 819–822.

15. Gardner, M.J., Hall, A.J., Snee, M.P., Downes, S., Powell, C.A. & Terrell, J.D. (1990). Methods and basic data of case-control study of leukaemia and lymphoma among young people near Sellafield nuclear plant in West Cumbria. *British Medical Journal*, 300, 429–434.

16. Gardner, M.J., Snee, M.P., Hall, A.J., Powell, C.A., Downes, S. & Terrell, J.D. (1990). Results of case-control study of leukaemia and lymphoma among young people near Sellafield nuclear plant in West Cumbria. *British Medical Journal*, 300, 423–429.

17 Nomura, T. (1982). Parental exposure to X-rays and chemicals induces heritable tumours and anomalies in mice. *Nature*, 296, 575–577.

18. Kinlen, L.J., Clarke, K. & Hudson, C. (1990). Evidence from population mixing in British New Towns 1946–85 of an infective basis for childhood leukaemia. *Medical Science*, 336, 577–582.

19. Alexander, F.E., Ricketts, T.J., McKinney, P.A. & Cartwright, R.A. (1990). Community lifestyle characteristics and risk of acute lymphoblastic leukaemia in children. *Lancet*, 336, 1461–1465.

20. Cook-Mozaffari, P., Darby, S.C. & Doll, R. (1989). Cancer near potential sites of nuclear installations. *Lancet*, ii, 1145–1147.

21. Hill, C. & Laplanche, A. (1990). Overall mortality and cancer mortality around French nuclear sites, *Nature*, 347, 755–757.

22. Jablon, S., Hrubec, Z., Boice, J.D. & Stone, B.J. (1990). *Cancer in Populations Living near Nuclear Facilities, Volumes 1, II and III*. NIH Publication No. 90–874. Washington: National Institutes of Health.

Gaia and Health

Public Health (1993), 107, 223–234. © The Society of Public Health, 1993, 9th Duncan Memorial Lecture, University of Liverpool, November 1991. J. Porritt. Thornbury House, 18 High Street, Cheltenham, Glos GL50 1DZ. Correspondence to: Mr J. Porritt.

As I did my preparatory work for this Lecture, and read through the learned contributions of my illustrious predecessors, I began to feel an ever stronger affinity with the work and example of William Duncan. Indeed, I have come to the conclusion that environmentalists and public health activists are simply different horses from the same stable, facing similar challenges – albeit in different races.

So wherein lie the similarities between environmentalists and public health activists? Environmentalists are concerned about the workings of Planet Earth, about identifying and analysing any damage to or breakdown of the different life-support systems on which we and all life forms depend. They are concerned (for the most part!) to minimise their own impact on the environment by a combination of consumer and lifestyle choices. They worry a lot, are prone to guilt, know very little about their antecedents, care about the interests of future generations, often have vaguely pagan feelings about the Earth itself, and eat a lot of fibre.

They share one further, all-important attribute: a presumption in both theory and practice in favour of prevention. For environmentalists, *post hoc* curative environmental policies (even successful ones) are a sign of a system's failure and of political immaturity. We can, for instance, clean up almost all of the tens of thousands of waste sites in Europe contaminated with toxic materials. The different treatment systems (engineering, chemical, biological) are increasingly ingenious and effective, but they are very costly. It would have been better by far if the damage could have been prevented in the first place by creating our wealth in such a way that it avoided such a devastating legacy.

For public health activists, *post hoc* curative responses to medical problems are often a sign of a systems failure or distorted economic and social priorities. The medicine of the 'magic bullet' is impressive, often extremely effective, but very costly. More often than not it would have been better by far to prevent the damage by taking a different approach to individual and community health.

Please do not read this as some iconoclastic, neo-Luddite knee jerk against modern technology. Having engendered such horrendous environmental and health costs, one can only be thankful that we are able very often to do something to mitigate or remove them – and there are many things for which any amount of preventive care will remain ineffective. But the grotesque imbalance in resource allocation, starving preventive health systems and sustainable wealth creation systems, is an aberration that should no longer be countenanced.

But it will be, of course, for some time to come. Current expenditure on preventive and community health care amounts to a minute proportion of the total health budget. Politicians in all the mainstream parties talk mindlessly of the need for increased expenditure on health, year after year after year. Parliamentary debates and the election exchanges are richly larded with competitive claims about entirely the wrong indicators of success: the number of operations; the number of outpatient treatments; the number of nurses and doctors employed and hospital beds filled. The more there are of each of these, the greater the degree of success claimed by respective political parties.

The sicker we are, it would seem, the greater the degree of success. As Thomas McKeown said, 'The disposal of society's investment in health is based on strange premises. It is assumed that we are ill and made well, whereas it is nearer to the truth that we are well and made ill'.[1]

So have today's politicians and experts simply stopped thinking, or are we truly insane? Even when they take a few tentative steps in the right direction, 50 years of arguing that more must necessarily be better has left politicians incapable of mapping out a new direction for our impossible overstretched illness services. Both the new arrangements for GPs and the separation of the roles of providers and purchasers of health services could become the building blocks of a new public health strategy that would revolutionise attitudes to health over the next few years. But even after the initial unpopularity that these measures have caused, government ministers still seem incapable of articulating clearly the potential within them. And their Labour shadows seem incapable of anything other than reflex rejection.

I suppose we should never underestimate the extent to which 250 years of industrialism have debilitated the human intellect and eroded the human spirit. For the last 20 years I have sat and listened to industrialists and politicians lecturing me about the need for permanent exponential growth in the economy: if we are not getting richer, they tell me, we will not have enough money to spend on cleaning up the environmental damage caused in the process of creating wealth.

Likewise, we are told that if we are not getting richer through permanent exponential growth in the economy, we will not have enough money to spend on the health service. Disregard the inconvenient fact that a lot of the ill health in industrial societies arises from the way we create wealth in the first place, the uses to which we put that wealth, and the inequitable distribution of that wealth. Those are merely the reformable 'malfunctions' of an intrinsically sound system.

'Rhubarb', say the environmentalists and public health activists. They are rather symptoms of an inherently distorted and distorting wealth creation system in which people have been persuaded that all human needs can best be met simply by increasing levels of production and consumption.

We have a long way to go before we are likely to overcome that prevailing orthodoxy.

People simply do not want to read the signs for what they tell us. We are facing massive infrastructural collapse on an almost unimaginable scale. The physical infrastructure of the Earth is under increasing strain from more and more people demanding more and more of both its finite non-renewable resources and its renewable resources (such as topsoil and forests) and services (such as pollution absorption). The physical and social infrastructure of our industrial economies is also under increasing strain from years of under-investment in maintenance and new systems. It is instructive, if a little depressing, to tot up the sums of money that independent analysts tell us should now be invested in new infrastructure for education, health, transport, sewage, housing, urban renewal, old age, disability and so on. No government on Earth could deliver – so why do they go on promising that they can? And why do we go on believing them, averting our eyes from the writing on the wall?

Infrastructure maintenance and replacement is one of the 'lost issues' of modern politics. The more capitalist society has accumulated in achieving exponential economic growth, the more there is either to maintain or to replace after depreciation. Hence the less there will be the year after, unless the inflow of new capital is enough to replace that which has been depreciated. Likewise, the more infrastructure there is, the higher the annual maintenance charge will be. Growth becomes a necessity (regardless of its desirability), simply to cover those service charges.

Unfortunately, we are all the victims of a singularly ill-informed debate about the nature and implications of economic growth. In particular, people are very confused about the significance of exponential economic growth.

> A quantity grows exponentially when its increase is proportional to what is already there. A colony of yeast cells in which each cell divides into two every ten minutes is growing exponentially. For each single cell after ten minutes there will be two cells. After the next ten minutes there will be four cells, ten minutes later there will be eight, then sixteen, and so on. The more yeast cells there are, the more new ones can be made. And that is exponential growth, doubling and redoubling and doubling again. Nearly everyone is surprised by it, because most people think linearly and think of growth as a linear process. A quantity grows linearly when it increases by a constant amount in a constant time period.[2]

The above extract may help to explain why environmentalists feel so concerned about the inability of politicians and electorates alike to understand the potential impact of people demanding permanent increases in rates of economic growth. They go on to give an even clearer example:

> There is an old Persian legend about a clever courtier who presented a beautiful chessboard to his king and requested that the king give him in

exchange one grain of rice for the first square on the board, two grains for the second square, four grains for the third, and so forth.

The king readily agreed, and ordered rice to be brought from his stores. The fourth square on the chessboard required eight grains, the tenth square took 512 grains, the fifteenth required 16,384 and the 21st square gave the courtier more than a million grains of rice. By the fortieth square a million million rice grains had to be piled up. The payment could never have continued to the 64th square; it would have taken more rice than there was in the whole world.[2] Given the quasi-mystical aura that surrounds the whole notion of economic growth, even some environmentalists have ceased to question its ineffectiveness as a policy tool as rigorously as they were once wont to do.

Theoretically, economic growth is the measure of increased economic activity in any one year. And theoretically at least, that is all it is; but rather than acknowledging the somewhat humble limitations to the concept and pursuit of economic growth, almost all politicians since the Second World War have progressively built up its conceptual significance so that, instead of it being one of the means by which we achieve our ends, it has become the single most important end of human society

The process is somewhat akin to obsessive obesity: instead of being a means to assuaging hunger, providing energy, ensuring convivial company or pleasant aesthetic experiences, the business of eating for such obsessives becomes the only activity which provides any kind of meaning or satisfaction or fulfilment. Eating itself becomes the goal of their existence. All industrial economies are now terminally confused between means and ends, between eating for living and eating for eating's sake.

Economic growth is simply not up to measuring economic welfare. It gives no indication of the sustainability of growth, and cannot measure the genuine efficiency of growth. Furthermore, it cannot indicate just who is benefiting from the growth, and cannot even discriminate between the genuine benefits of industrial production and the costs incurred in the process. Sadly, we are trapped by our own dependency on economic growth, not as a means to an end, but as an end in itself – indeed almost as a new godhead, before which we all dutifully genuflect. Every conceivable subterfuge and intellectual dishonesty is engaged in by politicians to avoid having to come to terms with this uncomfortable truth. Scientific evidence about the direct impact of exponential growth on our life-support systems (with more people inexorably demanding more from a strictly finite resource base and pollution absorption capacity) is dismissed as temporary or of secondary importance. If sustainability is to be the key economic concept of the future, then the use of Gross National Product (GNP) as the exclusive measure of economic success has obviously had its day. It is a bit like trying to assess one's enjoyment of a piece of music by measuring the number of notes in it! Or, as Edward Abbey put it rather more succinctly, 'growth for the sake of growth is the ideology of the cancer cell'.

Such a medical analogy is not inappropriate. For there are few indicators that more accurately reflect the real well-being of people than the state of their health. Between 1955 and 1988, GNP per head in the UK doubled; in theory, all citizens were at that moment twice as rich as their parents had been at the same time. You might reasonably suppose that in the same 33-year period, all citizens were getting progressively healthier, if not exactly twice as healthy.

In one respect, you would be right. Most infectious diseases have become far less prevalent and life expectancy at all ages has improved. But if you looked at other indicators, you would come to a very different conclusion.

> According to the Government's General Household Survey for 1988, thirty three per cent of the population had a long-standing illness that year, up from twenty one per cent in 1972, and whereas only eight per cent of those interviewed in 1971 had reported being acutely ill during the preceding weeks, in 1988, fourteen per cent did. Similarly, the average number of days for which the state paid out sickness and invalidity benefits to each insured worker rose from 8.8 in 1962 to 12.2 in 1988. Again, 226 million prescriptions – 4.7 per head – were issued in 1961, when they were free, and newspapers complained that spongers were using them to obtain items as cheap and trivial as bottles of aspirin; in 1988, the number was 427.7 million – 7.5 per person – despite the deterrent of a £2.60 charge. In addition, hospital admissions almost doubled, and would have been higher still had the health service been able to cope.[3]

Richard Wilkinson of the Trafford Centre for Medical Research at the University of Sussex has studied the link between patterns of ill health and income levels since the mid-1970s. He believes that the relationship between income distribution and health is absolutely clear; indeed, he has stated that about two-thirds of the variation in life expectancy between different countries is related to differences in their income distribution:

> Since the early 1970s, Japan has gone from the middle of the field in terms of life expectancy and income distribution to the top in both. Japan now has the highest recorded life expectancy and the most egalitarian income distribution in the world. On the other side of the coin, while Britain's income distribution worsened dramatically during the Eighties to produce the largest inequalities for over a century, its relative position in terms of life expectancy has also worsened. Each year since 1985 mortality rates among both men and women between the ages of sixteen and forty-five have actually risen – a trend which is not attributable to death from AIDS.[4]

It is one thing to demonstrate increased patterns of ill health during a period of prolonged economic growth. It is quite another to demonstrate cause and effect. This has not yet been done. But as the evidence builds up about dietary patterns (particularly the excessive consumption of sugar), of food additives, pesticides, air pollution in general (and heavy metals and volatile organic compounds in particular), radiation and electric magnetic pollution, and a host of other 'environmental factors', somewhere down the line someone is going to be able not just to assert but definitively to prove the connection between ill health and the aggregated by-products of the pursuit of exponential economic growth.

In the meantime, uncertainty and ignorance continue to underpin today's unethical and unsustainable system of wealth creation. Uncertainty continues to allow politicians to argue that there is 'insufficient evidence' to justify any policy development or new pattern of expenditure. Ignorance bolsters unhealthy lifestyles. The average man or woman on a Clapham omnibus remains hopeless at making any kind of personal risk assessment. No amount of mind-numbing statistical information about the impact of smoking on people's health has proved sufficient to free millions from their habit or even to stop millions of young people from taking it up.

And how long will be required to reverse two decades of sun-worshipping vanity now that there is no serious scientific dispute about the dangers of ozone depletion? One thousand people die of skin cancer in the UK every year. The incidence of melanoma in Scotland rose by 82% between 1979 and 1989; researchers claim that cases are doubling every eight years for men and every 13 years for women. But, despite all that, recent surveys in America have revealed, almost unbelievably, that the majority of parents still believe that a suntanned skin is an indicator of good health in their children.

Such problems of education and persuasion are of course not new. Indeed, did not William Duncan face exactly the same kind of resistance arising in part out of ignorance and in part out of the defence of vested interest? As Sidney Chave said (in the Inaugural Lecture in this series):

> But the idea of a medical police was not to the taste of the English with their 'Victorian values', where *laissez-faire*, sturdy independence, and unfettered private enterprise was the accepted dogma. Only gradually, under the unanswerable case of state intervention to control private interests in favour of the public weal, did this characteristically English philosophy begin to break down.[5]

For all the great advances we have made in science and technology, we hardly seem to have made equivalent strides in human wisdom. I sometimes think that the precautionary principle is no less subordinated to a 'where is the pile of bodies' approach to medicine now that it was in Duncan's day! But the point is that he really did have the bodies to hand to prove his case; hardly surprising with an annual death rate in Liverpool in 1840 of 36 per thousand – the highest in the country.

There are, of course, many parts of the world where the bodies are already piled high enough even for the most doubting of Thomases. An audience like this will be all too familiar with the statistics of Third World suffering, but I suspect that even such an audience will have developed defence mechanisms against the pain that this might otherwise cause them or the moral dilemmas that it persistently raises. We all know that the rich are getting richer and the poor are getting poorer, but whatever happened to the contradictory impulse set in train by Band Aid?

The burden of international debt on Third World countries provides a telling example of how we have developed appropriate defence mechanisms. The debt service ratio (the proportion of GNP a country has to devote to paying off its debts) is one of the most telling indicators of both national and individual prosperity. Many Third World countries today see more than 40% of GNP disappear on debt repayments, and no amount of new and additional funding will help lift that crushing burden. The net transfer of around 50 billion dollars per annum from South to North (made up mostly of debt repayments) provides the most abhorrent reminder of just what happens when the world is handed over to bankers.

A programme of comprehensive debt relief (of both government and private sector debt) would be the single most effective way of helping Third World countries to meet the challenge of sustainable development. But most people refuse to acknowledge their own personal involvement in that process, notwithstanding the fact that it is to their own friendly high street bank that these debts are owed.

The 'Big Four' high street banks are currently owed more than £9 billion by debtor countries in the Third World. The human suffering that is incurred in efforts to repay those debts is of course appalling, but what makes it all the worse is the manoeuvring that surrounds it.

Let us start with tax relief. Bankers believe that much of the debt will never be repaid. So they set aside part of their annual profits as 'provisions' against those bad debts. In its wisdom, the government then allows them tax relief on those provisions; to date, the banks have retained more than £1.6 billion that they would otherwise have paid in tax. You can build quite a few hospitals or employ a lot of teachers with £1.6 billion.

But with most people indifferent to the suffering of those whose environment has already collapsed and as yet unconvinced that their own environment is under threat of collapse, what realistic chance do we have of effecting a sufficiently rapid and thoroughgoing transformation of the world economy to rescue us from the worst consequences of our abuse of the Earth? Many of my colleagues subscribe somewhat fatalistically to the view that it will only get better once it has got worse, that intimations of apocalypse must be seared personally and painfully into our minds before the need for radical change is openly acknowledged.

For some, AIDS already fits that particular bill. Professor Roy Anderson, Head of Biology at Imperial College, believes that in some countries in Africa the HIV virus will eventually kill far more people every year than will be born, thus reversing decades of population growth. In the worst afflicted areas of Africa, the virus is already afflicting more than 30% of pregnant women.

There remains considerable controversy about such predictions; the Overseas Development Administration (ODA), for example, believes that the plateau in the incidence of AIDS will be reached at a level well below that associated with population decline. But at least all experts agree on one thing: the idea that AIDS might help to relieve hunger by reducing population is an absolute myth. And a dangerous one at that.

AIDS kills off those between 15 and 50, the most economically active in any population, and leaves the very young and very old to try and cover the gap. A recent paper from the World Bank on the effects of AIDS on economic productivity in Africa predicts a 22% decline in Gross Domestic Product in a typical African country. Biologists have also pointed out that when human numbers double or even triple (to 16/17 billion), our species will then become so numerous as to be an environment in itself. Our bodies will become the stamping ground for the inevitable proliferation of new viruses. And it is worth bearing in mind that we already use for our own ends more than 40% of the planet's net terrestrial photosynthesis. Twice as many of us may well lay claim to 80%, with terrifying consequences for the erosion of today's genetic diversity.

AIDS has been described as nature's revenge on humankind. Gaia strikes back against humanity's cancerous growth. I find such metaphors disturbing, but they may serve to sharpen our perception of the way in which the planet works. It is now 20 years since Jim Lovelock and Lyn Margulis first put forward their Gaia hypothesis, postulating the idea of the Earth as a self-regulating super organism, a single physiological system.[6] Lovelock describes Gaia as something like an oven thermostat, maintaining its chemistry and temperature at levels optimal for the sustaining of life on Earth. He makes no claim, by the way, that this is a purposeful process.

This challenging hypothesis continues to perturb the scientific establishment, which is accustomed to process life through the rather narrow filters of their specialist disciplines. But if the Earth is indeed one single system, it must be unhelpful to keep on separating it up into categories such as biosphere, atmosphere, lithosphere and hydrosphere. These are merely the academic pigeonholes in which people compete amongst themselves for promotional research budgets; they provide a wholly inaccurate template for the workings of the Earth.

Lovelock draws a comparison here between contemporary specialised medicine and the older (in his view, more honourable) profession of physiology. He believes it is now crucial to develop a new generation of planetary physicians to help us overcome the limitations of narrow focus microbiologists or geochemists or a host of other specialisms (Table I).

Table I: Tools and methods in human and planetary medicine

Measurement	Human	Planet
Temperature	Clinical thermometer	Satellite radiometer
Blood pressure	Sphygmomanometer	Barometer
Breathing	Stethoscope	Atmospheric carbon dioxide monitors
Biochemical tests	Blood and urine samples	Air and sea samples
Biopsy	Tissue samples	Ecosystem studies

Source: Lovelock, J. (1991). *Gaia: The Practical Science of Planetary Medicine*. Gaia Books.

It if is true that we are suffering from a series of planetary diseases (of which AIDS is just as likely to be a symptom as ozone depletion), then we need planetary medical advice without further delay. Diagnosticians such as Paul Ehrlich, Teddy Goldsmith and Lester Brown have been hard at work for decades. Countless prescriptions have been prepared, but never taken up. Lovelock extends his medical analogy by reference to the likes of Chadwick and Duncan:

> In the last century, the environmental problems were just as serious as our own today. In the mid nineteenth century, there were epidemics of the waterborne diseases, cholera and typhoid, that caused the death of a third of the inhabitants of some cities in a few months. Science was not then organised as a powerful lobby, and was prepared to admit that it did not know the cause of the diseases. Physicians at the sharp end of this battle suspected from the epidemiology that infection was waterborne or came from the bad odours of the primitive sewage systems then in use. But our practical forebears did not pour funds into the infant science of microbiology and wait until it was proved that cholera and typhoid were waterborne bacterial infections. They acted promptly and empirically by installing clean water supplies and efficient sewage collection and disposal plants. Engineering was in those days a proud profession, and triumphantly displayed its self-confidence in those amazing Gothic pumping stations that are now a place of pilgrimage for students of industrial architecture.[7]

Lovelock's theory of planetary medicine may sound rather too grand and global for the hands-on empiricists of today's public health movement! But it translates easily and conveniently into a whole series of admirably practical policies, both for individuals and the whole National Health Service. As we all know, our sickness services are not exactly models of environment-friendly behaviour, and a disturbingly large number of people end up sicker as a direct consequence of seeking treatment for their original sickness.

Even on basics, the National Health Service is something of an ecological horror story. The National Association of Waste Disposal Contractors have shown that most of the 800 incinerators used by Health Authorities in the UK cannot burn waste at the required temperature, causing high levels of pollutants such as heavy metals, dioxins, acids and sulphur to be emitted. Hospital incinerators are not checked by Her Majesty's Inspectorate of Pollution, nor are environmental health officers obliged to check emissions.

The National Audit Office produced a report in 1991 showing that the National Health Service could cut its energy consumption by at least 15%, saving £30 million in the process.[8] It suggested that energy efficiency targets should be included when assessing performance pay for hospital managers. If performance-related pay is to remain all the rage, then let the performance be as much about achieving high environmental standards as saving money.

I could go on. The challenge to health professionals to sort out their own house is enormous. But are these not more propitious times for achieving higher environmental performance through increased efficiency? Cost saving and getting value for money need not always penalise the patient or health practitioner. At long last, government ministers are beginning to talk rather more intelligently about health promotion strategies rather than curative responses. The Government's White Paper, *The Health of the Nation*,[9] is a genuinely welcome breakthrough inasmuch as the setting of hard targets (to reduce heart diseases and strokes in people under 65, to reduce smoking, cut fat consumption and encourage exercise) creates the context in which resource allocation decisions within the National Health Service must now be taken. It is of course utterly daft to seek to reduce smoking while simultaneously refusing to ban all cigarette advertising, but the tobacco lobby still knows how to serve its own interests by lobbying government ministers effectively.

Health promotion and preventive medicine are decidedly on the up again in policy circles. The World Health Organisation strategy of Health for All by the Year 2000, as well as the Healthy Cities project, have done much to legitimise that shift in emphasis. But public perception still lags someway behind thinking within the policy community. As David Player has pointed out:

> To most health consumers, the professions involved in public health normally appear on the dark side of the health moon. While the treatment services are bathed in publicity, glamour and some notoriety, the people responsible for sanitation, food hygiene and catering, safety at work, pollution monitoring, control of epidemics and other preventive measures hit media high spots only over failure in their performance as preventers and watchdogs.

That is certainly true, but even this may be changed by another important philosophical shift that has taken place over the last few years. We have seen a move away from old-fashioned 'clientism', in which individuals abrogated responsibility for their own health, and health professionals tried to fill the role of omniscient if not omnipotent deliverers of good health. An intriguing convergence has emerged between the Conservative Party's emphasis on individualism and personal responsibility and the resurgence of complementary or holistic alternatives to orthodox medicine. The Left continues to feel uneasy about this move away from a collectivised and standardised health care system, but a more flexible, individually tailored approach, stressing personal lifestyle rather than dependence on the magic bullet, is undoubtedly more in keeping with the spirit of the times. It just happens to be more in keeping with Green philosophy as well. As John Ashton points out, 'The concept of reciprocal maintenance – that we should look after the things that look after us – is rapidly gathering ground, whether those things are our own bodies or the planet itself.[10]

Not that this for one moment detracts from the hugely important work that still has to be done demonstrating the link between poverty and ill health. Though the Government's White Paper studiously attempts to ignore those connections, there is no getting round the evidence of the Black report[11] or other studies which show that the substantial increase in the numbers of people on or below the poverty line over the last 12 years has had an extremely damaging impact on the nation's health. The more callous aspects of this Government's 'Devil take the hindmost, survival of the fittest' philosophy render all but null and void its new-found enthusiasm for prevention and health promotion. You cannot promote health by systematically impoverishing ever larger numbers of people in order to go on enriching a few.

And was this not precisely the message that William Duncan sought to get across to his audiences and in his evidence to the Chadwick enquiry? The *laissez-faire* absolutism of his age has many resonances with the free market monetarism of our own.

But reality has a way of creeping back into the pores of any political process; current statistics about increases in wealth differentials and poverty are going to prove a great deal harder for Mr Major to ignore than they were for Mrs Thatcher. In exactly the same way, statistics about the state of the Earth and the crushing burden of misery for millions of people in the Third World are already transforming the climate of opinion about appropriate policy responses. It remains a frustratingly slow business persuading politicians to accept that evidence, but the United Nations Conference on Environment and Development in June 1992 marked a watershed in terms of international acknowledgement of the state of the Earth, even if it failed ultimately in putting in place as many of the answers as it should have.

Two key phrases run through the various documents produced at the Rio Earth Summit: sustainable development and the precautionary principle. On the virtues of sustainable development, there would now seem to be overwhelming international consensus. Indeed, one might ask how we could have ever countenanced development models that could only be delivered by denying the rights of future generations to an equitable share in the world's finite natural wealth. True enough, we are still a million miles away from actually achieving anything like sustainable development, but the idea that this generation should seek to meet its needs and improve its quality of life 'within the carrying capacity of the planet and in ways that are not detrimental to future generations' remains a hugely important conceptual breakthrough.

The precautionary principle may come to assume an equal significance. For it implicitly acknowledges the limitations of our scientific and technological prowess. A little humility does at last seem to be tempering the white-hot fervour of the modern scientific establishment. And that is not really so surprising, given that the more we discover about the workings of the Earth, the more we discover how little we actually know. In circumstances of continuing uncertainty or ignorance, the emphasis must therefore be on caution and restraint rather than on bravado gestures and the pursuit of perceptible 'progress' for its own sake.

Arguably, we are somewhat better informed about the workings of the human body. We can certainly be in no doubt that the precautionary principle is of equal significance here as in matters planetary. Historically, it has of course been the public health movement that has upheld the precautionary principle since the time of Chadwick and Duncan. But, as an outsider, I cannot help thinking that the profession now needs to evaluate how best to carry out that role in a very different world. And it was no less an authority than John Ashton who put the challenge to his own colleagues in a BMJ editorial back in January 1991:

> Over many decades, the work of public health pioneers has been defined and codified, frozen in relation to another era and another way of looking at the world. Its practice now seems to have become reactive and bureaucratic, rather than pro-active and innovative. Practitioners of the new public health need to have a good grounding in the ecology and the vision of how to reconcile the natural and the built environment. They need to revisit all the topics of the old public health – housing, food, water, sanitation, education, occupation, transport, genetics and microbiology, and medical and social services – and to re-examine them with ecological eyes. This has considerable implications for the education and training and for the work patterns of those who work in public health, not least for those whose roots lie in environmental health. There is, particularly, a need for new multi-disciplinary initiatives in both training and working.[12]

And that kind of re-evaluation would seem to be going on here as much as anywhere else in the country. It simply is not enough to fall back on the good old cliché about 'a healthy mind in a healthy body'. For we cannot expect to find healthy human bodies on a sick planet. The true challenge in green politics is to persuade people once and for all that the wounds we inflict on the Earth we inflict also on ourselves. Just as holistic medicine seeks to address itself to the whole human entity (mind, body and spirit), so holistic green politics seeks to address itself to the inextricable interconnectedness of life on Earth.

The concept of interdependence is not some whimsical product of Guardian-reading romantics. It emerges from hard empirical data about the life-support systems on which we all depend. Sceptics and realists alike continue to argue that, with human nature being what it is, interdependence will remain forever the provenance of unwordly Greens. But I would dispute the argument that we will never save the Earth unless we first manage a complete transformation of human nature. It is, after all, only very recently that we have chosen to ignore and even become ashamed of our evolutionary antecedents. That process of evolution provides as many examples of cooperation as it does of competition, and though it is true that we now stand apart from the rest of life on Earth in several critical respects, we are still very much a part of it and utterly dependent on it, whether we like it or not.

But at the very least, we shall have to reinterpret the notion of self-interest. Was it not ever thus! To refer again to Sidney Chave's inaugural lecture in this series (from which you can see that I have learned a great deal!), he quoted from a Dr Liddle, the Medical Officer of Health for Whitechapel in the mid-nineteenth century:

It cannot be too often impressed upon our minds that sickness among the poor is the great cause of pressure upon the rates. In the course of time, the public will learn that sickness with its concomitant evils – loss of wages, calls upon clubs and friendly societies, the increased amount of charitable contributions, a heavier poll rate, entails more expense upon the community than would be required to carry out sanitary improvements in widening streets and in erecting more commodious houses for the poor.[5]

It was then (as people like Dr Liddle and William Duncan recognised only too well), as it still is today, folly to suppose that we can supplant self-interest as the dominant motivating factor in people's lives. But we can enrich it, deepen it and breathe new life into it by dissolving some of the artificial dividing lines between 'the self' (as interpreted in its narrowest series) and the rest of life on Earth.

We are all, to varying degrees, trapped by images of our own power and superiority, by a centuries-old failure to balance our rights and entitlements as the dominant species on Earth with the all-important obligation to protect and value the rest of life on Earth for its own sake, and not just for its usefulness to us.

True enough, if we are indeed one strand in the web of life, then we are obviously unable to protect our species without simultaneously protecting the entire web. But a crudely utilitarian ethic ('protect it only if it benefits us') will ensure that we go on losing as many battles as we win. For who is to define 'usefulness'? Only if we ascribe intrinsic (though not necessarily equal) value to all life forms are we likely to find both the means and the collective political will to protect the living Earth on any kind of sustainable basis.

It was Archbishop William Temple who once wrote:

The treatment of the Earth by man the exploiter is not only imprudent, it is sacrilegious. We are not likely to correct our hideous mistakes in this realm unless we recover the mystical sense of our oneness with nature. Many people think this is fantastic. I think it is fundamental to our sanity.

If the self is at one with the rest of life on Earth, then self-interest takes on a very different meaning. And that for me is the challenge that lies at the heart of 'planetary medicine' today, and the common ground on which environmentalists and public health activists should gather to launch another (hopefully final!) assault on the bastions of modern medical and political orthodoxy.

References

1. McKeown, T. (1988). *The Origins of Human Disease*. Oxford: Blackwell.
2. Meadows, D. H., Meadows, D. L. & Randers, J. (1992). *Beyond the Limits: Global Collapse or Sustainable Future*, p. 17. London: Earthscan.
3. Douthwaite, R. (1992), *The Growth Illusion*. London: Resurgence Books.
4. Wilkinson, R. G (1990). Income distribution and mortality: a 'natural' experiment. *Sociology of Health and Illness*, 12(4), 391–412.

5. Chave, S. P. W. (1984). Duncan of Liverpool – and Some Lessons for Today. *Community Medicine*, 6(1), 61–71.
6. Lovelock, J. (1991), *Gaia: The Practical Science of Planetary Medicine*. Gaia Books.
7. Lovelock, J., ibid, p. 14.
8. National Audit Office (1991). *NHS Outpatient Services*. HC191, 1990/91. London: HMSO.
9. Department of Health (1991). *The Health of the Nation*. London: Department of Health.
10. Ashton, J. & Seymour, H. (1988). The New Public Health. Milton Keynes: Open University Press.
11. Black, D. A. K., Townsend, P. & Davidson, N. (1982). *Inequalities in Health – the Black Report*. Harmondsworth: Penguin.
12. Ashton, J. (1991). Sanitarian becomes ecologist: the new environmental health. *British Medical Journal*, (26 January) 302, 189–190.

Prospects for Public Health in Europe after 1992

Duncan Memorial Lecture, University of Liverpool, December 9, 1992.
Dr Robert Anderson.

Introduction

This paper will focus upon international action to promote the public's health, and specifically will concentrate upon the role and contribution of the institutions of the European Community. It aims to demonstrate how the EC is already engaged in a variety of initiatives that are important for public health; secondly to argue that the EC's involvement in public health matters is likely to increase substantially; and finally to propose that with the active, informed participation of public and professionals the prospects for public health after 1992 can be improved through action at EC level.

Before this, though, it is customary to reflect upon the pioneering contribution of Dr (William Henry) Duncan. The Single European Act is designed to promote the movement of goods, services and people. In his work Dr. Duncan was critically exposed to the effects of population movements. The middle years of the last century witnessed the migration of poor and starved Irish people, as well as others from Germany and the Netherlands, into some of the worst imaginable and crowded housing conditions in Liverpool. The epidemics confronted by Duncan appear to have been triggered by this migration. The migration of populations, from outside and between countries of the EC, often deprived and looking for employment, is likely to be an increasingly important feature and factor strongly influencing public health in Europe. It will be stimulated in part by legal and other initiatives in the EC.

I should also like to refer to Duncan's use of international comparison in his small canon of published work. He ended his lectures to the Literary and Philosophical Society in 1843 by comparing the status and place of public health in this country unfavourably with that in 'France and other continental countries'. This sensitivity to experience elsewhere, and the rather direct comparison of data from different countries has been, and continues to be, an important stimulus to research and action in public health.

The series of 1992 articles in the British Medical Journal on 'Medicine in Europe' begins by considering why it is that middle aged men and women in Britain are three times as likely to die from coronary heart disease as their counterparts in France. The very substantial differences between Member States of the EC – for example, in mortality from coronary heart disease and stroke

– stimulate questions about causation, but also strengthen demands for action on the grounds that 'we can do better'. In particular, differences in health and illness experiences by country (and also consistently where data exist by gender and social class) give rise to questions about the place of intervention by the different public health and health care systems. In some ways these different systems constitute 'natural experiments' – a basis for comparison and learning between Member States, but within the EC institutions they also offer the potential for improved, more effective and efficient, co-operation.

I will turn now to review developments for public health in the EC, particularly in relation to the Single European Act which was signed in 1986 and came into force in July 1987; and then specifically consider potential implications of the Maastricht Treaty, if and when it is ratified.

Public health in the EC

European Community Ministers of Health have been meeting since 1977, although only since 1986 has this been as frequently a twice a year. This reflects the economic focus of the 1957 Treaty of Rome, which hardly mentions, and therefore gives little priority to action for, health.

There are Articles in the founding Treaty about improving living and working conditions, assurance of social security or workers, and health protection. The last has been amplified in the Single European Act Article 118A, which emphasises safety and health of workers. This focus on health and safety of workers is the main thrust of EC health policy; elsewhere health is a marginal issue. There is no focal point for health matters in the European Communities. It is a subject of several Directorates General (effectively small ministries or departments), notably DG V (Social Affairs) which covers occupational health and safety as well as the emerging interest in public health. A small public health unit was established in 1988, based, like the other Health and Safety units, in Luxembourg. Directorate-General XII has responsibility for a growing research programme while DG VI deals with the quality and safety of agricultural products. The Consumer Policy Service reviews the labelling and safety of products while health issues arise peripherally in the remits of at least five other DG's, such as Transport and Environment. It has certainly been argued that there has been a lack of communication and co-ordination between Director-ate-Generals on health matters. Furthermore they have generally worked with small administrative staffs. However, numbers and health-related expertise of both the Public Health and Health Research units have increased in the last five years, reflecting increased priority given by Member States to some health issues.

While steps towards the Single European Market in 1992 do not include integration or harmonisation of the health and social security systems the EC is engaged in a wide range of actions (seldom legislation) more or less relevant to health.

Current EC actions

In the last decade several issue-oriented initiatives have been launched, all at the specific request of the Council of Health Ministers rather than as elements of concerted policies or mandated programmes. Although such one-off initiatives give profile and some funds for public health they are not part of any comprehensive health strategy. This makes their profile and funding vulnerable to changes in political commitment. Most of these have been coordinated through Directorate General V (Social Affairs). The main initiatives are: 'Europe Against Cancer' established in 1985 to promote research, information, public awareness and training of relevant personnel. It is mainly directed at individual action for the prevention of cancer. The 'Action Against Tobacco' initiative deals with advertising, tobacco products, taxation, and pricing policies. Unfortunately, these initiatives have funds that are insignificant compared with the amounts spent each year to subsidise tobacco production in the EC. 'Action Against Drugs' is directed towards information provision and education to prevent drug abuse, as well as exchange of information on the treatment and social integration of drug addicts. A programme to combat AIDS looks at prevention, coping with the impacts, and coordination of international activities. Like the recent Council Resolution on 'nutrition and health', these initiatives are typical of the Commission's action programmes, concentrating, as they do, on support for pilot projects, exchanges of information and development of research.

The Commission gives support to initiatives designed to improve the quality of life of disadvantaged groups, but views health care as clearly the responsibility of Member States. The main and direct health initiative in the Commission deals with measures for the protection of workers, and this has been substantially extended as a consequence of the Single European Act (SEA).

Health research supported by the Commission has been driven largely by the economic concerns of the health care industry and health care providers. There has been a relatively small programme of health services research which appears to have made little impact on health system policy makers in member States. The SEA emphasises the need to generate a better balance between economic and social development, and gave a real boost to research – essentially to improve co-ordination and more efficient use of resources (human and financial). The importance of medically oriented research appears to be rising, with the establishment of 'Biomed 1' funded with 133 million ECU as the flagship of the EC's biomedical and health research (1990–94). This is still only 2.3% of the total research budget and, of course, tiny as a proportion of national research funds and this sum must be divided between 12 countries over five years). The main areas in this programme are: the development of coordinated research on prevention, care and health systems; major health problems and diseases of great socio-economic impact (e.g. AIDS, cancer, cardiovascular disease, and mental illness); and Human Genome Analysis. A second programme of Advanced Informatics in Medicine has been allocated a budget of 97 million ECU for the same period – part of this budget is dedicated to the development of a European Health Care Information infrastructure taking into account the needs of users and technological opportunities. There is currently no comparable set of data on health and health care of the 12 Member States.

Direct effects of the Single European Act

Other than research, there appear to be relatively few direct effects of the Single European Act on health and health care. The clearest references are related to:

Occupational health and safety – the objective is to harmonise regulations on health and safety, taking as a base a high level of protection; and to encourage improvements to guarantee better levels of protection. The Directives include both a general framework for protecting the health of the whole working population, and a set of more specific initiatives for groups of workers such as VDU users, pregnant women and construction workers. This health and safety legislation may provide some basis for reviewing other aspects of the working environment or employment practices related to health.

Drugs – the White Paper, the schedule towards the Single European Market, includes 13 measures specifically directed to the pharmaceutical sector. By 1992 all industrially produced medicines will be covered through harmonisation of criteria for safety, quality and efficacy. A 1990 Directive provides for full transparency of price control measures for drugs paid for by national social security systems, allowing some right of appeal by industry. However, analysts do not expect this to lead to competitive pricing on an EC-wide basis. Overall, and given the substantial programme in the pharmaceutical sector there is a surprising lack of assessment of the impact of the new legislation. There are proposals for the establishment of a European Medicines Agency (possibly akin to the United States Food and Drug Administration).

Labour mobility – the general orientation of the SEA is to promote mobility of workers, as well as goods, services and capital, generating a more efficient allocation of scarce resources in Member States. In the health sector there has been a major drive over 15 years for mutual recognition of training, professional and educational qualifications. As of January 1991 mutual recognition was obtained for professional qualifications involving at least three years training for doctors, dentists, nurses, vets, pharmacists and midwives. There are concerns that there may not be full comparability between countries, reflecting, for example, skills and experience as well as academic qualifications. There are also open questions about language ability, and the familiarity of professionals with the health and social security systems in other Member States. The existing opportunities for employment mobility have been taken up by only a small minority; for example, it has been estimated only 12,000 out of 900,000 doctors (1.3%) practice in another Member State. There is little reason to expect that the new provisions of the Maastricht Treaty will dramatically increase mobility. Increased opportunities for practice in Member States may influence the distribution of staff to the extent that differences in salaries and conditions of service result in some staff moving between countries. High salary countries with staff shortages in specialised areas, such as paediatric cardiology nursing, may be able to attract such specialists from low salary countries on the basis of pay and conditions. Low salary countries may be forced to raise their pay levels to prevent loss of specialists. In the longer term, all pay differentials may have to be adjusted, leading to common European rates of pay (with only small local variations) for health care specialists. Increased professional mobility will also make more transparent variations in staffing levels and employment practices. This creates an opportunity to extend good practices more widely.

Single European Act – indirect effects

Considering less direct effects of the Single European Act, it must be acknowledged that the range of the Act is so extensive that almost any part of the health field could be affected. This reflects the general orientation of EC policy to achieve better living standards and working conditions across all Member States. From the range of possible impacts the following seem most pertinent to health:

Harmonisation of excise duties – specifically taxes on alcohol and tobacco which should be revised to a common level in all Member States. Since pricing policies are held to have an effect on consumption, it has been accepted that for health reasons excise duties should not go down, which might otherwise have been the case in some Member States. Also by 1992/3 the EC hopes to have harmonised the labelling of cigarette packets, with obligatory health warnings, to eliminate tax-free sales of cigarettes, and to prohibit cigarettes with a high tar content.

Health insurance – from January 1993 health insurance companies will be free to carry out business throughout the EC. This will have implications for cost competition between the providers of care, for cross-national transfers of patients and possibly for concentrations and vacuums in specific service provision. Multinational providers may concentrate some of their services in low cost, low wage countries. The result could be a flow of patients to Southern States. Alternatively, and probably more likely, there will be a flow of patients from countries such as Greece and Italy, to centres of excellence in the centre of the Community. The private insurance sector expects to grow and to benefit from SEA directives concerning the free movement of goods and services, and unhampered access to an integrated market. They may accelerate 'medical tourism' by offering a variety of packages, such as that to the 30 Danes each week who travel to recuperate in Malaga! Clearly, the Commission needs to monitor these developments in private health insurance to ensure that greater inequalities in access to care do not result.

It is possible that health care, as well as health issues, will become more internationalised. Patients may move (with their health card for emergencies), or be moved to receive treatment in places where it is cheaper or more readily available. There may be some improvement in general efficiency, and a relative reduction in health care costs.

Maastricht Treaty

In the SEA, public health is discussed in relation to the effects of increased migration and its control, e.g. with regard to infectious diseases. Now, with the Treaty revisions proposed in Maastricht, there is the prospect of much more fundamental change.

The Treaty on European Union, signed in Maastricht in February 1992 includes a new Article on Public Health. This gives the European Community, for the first time, an explicit mandate for public health. The new Article recognises that the health of people in Europe depends on much more than the provision of health care and health services. Since the health situation in one country will clearly affect conditions in other countries, there is an emphasis on the need to cooperate and coordinate activities between Member States, in order to combat the major causes of ill health.

The Treaty underlines the significance of co-operation with countries outside the Community, and with the competent international organisations in the sphere of public health. Article 129 on Public Health, which will be subject to qualified majority voting, emphasises the promotion of research, as well as health information and education. It focuses upon health promotion and disease prevention, and it recognises the need to consider health protection as a constituent part of the Community's other policies. It therefore offers the prospect of reviewing policies in agriculture, transport and environment for their potential impacts on health.

The Maastricht article leaves a lot unwritten such as the definition of public health and how major health scourges are to be conceived. They are certainly likely to include those issues on which the Council of Ministers has already established programmes – AIDS, cancer, alcohol, and specifically drug dependence. However two other categories are foreseeable: for action on diseases with a high rate of mortality; and for action on illnesses with a high impact on the quality of life, such as arthritis and mental illness.

In Conclusion

Perhaps the major strategic task for public health associated with the Maastricht agreement is to build up an awareness about health in Europe, both its distribution and determinants. There is a need to identify and implement interventions which bring about the maximum improvements in health, particularly for those groups in the population who are currently disadvantaged. Member States, regional and local units need information on health status and its distribution among the population as a basis for establishing priorities and local needs. Reliable and timely epidemiological data, such as population surveys and studies of health and lifestyles, are not available in many regions, and consequently not at all on a comparative basis for the Community as a whole.

The significance for health of public policies in sectors such as agriculture, industry, transport, energy and environment is widely acknowledged. The Community's commitment to considering health protection requirements as part of general policies is important. However there has been little systematic attention to such health impact assessment studies, nor is the methodology for such analysis well developed. Without such information the prospects for the development of coherent public health policy will be diminished.

There is now an opportune moment to promote better health in Europe and to strengthen public health. There is clearly a need for appropriate organisational structures to accomplish new tasks, particularly to assess the health impacts of other Community policies. A strong focal point is required to strengthen the development and dissemination of research. There is a need for some institutional base, not only for exchange and analysis of this research but also to share models of innovative practice. Much of the recent action to improve health emphasises the importance and initiative of citizen movements or consumer organisations. Other key allies for health in the Community include, of course, health, education and environment professionals, as well as the media, parliamentarians, local authorities, trade unions, and voluntary organisations.

The challenge for international bodies, but especially for the professional groups, is to develop mechanisms for communication at a European level. There is an urgent need to enhance links between these professional associations, and also for network-building to involve other citizen and representative organisations.

The EC can play an important, if limited, role in this strengthening of public health. Even if the pace of any legislation is likely to be slow, there are significant needs and opportunities to improve the quality and comparability of health information and analysis. In particular better co-operation and co-ordination between Member States can make it possible to complete achievements in the field of public health, contributing to exchange and implementation of improved policy and practice.

Who cares for health? Social relations, gender, and the public health

Journal of Epidemiology and Community Health (1994); 48:427–434.
Duncan memorial lecture. Ann Oakley. Social Science Research Unit,
University of London Institute of Education, 20 Bedford Way, London
WC1H 0AL. Presented at the University of Liverpool, 1 December 1993.

It is important to begin by thanking those who invited me to give this lecture, which will provide me with an opportunity to talk about all my favourite topics. You will be pleased to hear that I am able to trace some respectable historical antecedents in the field of public health. A paternal relation of mine was William Farr, statistician to Britain's first Registrar General. My father was Richard Titmuss, whose work in the late 1940s and early 1950s on class inequalities in health and illness jointly with Jerry Morris helped to shape the emerging discipline of social medicine.[1] Social medicine was closely related to the domain of public health, as is its successor, the sociology of health and illness.

But genetic credentials for talking about public health, or social medicine, or whatever one chooses to call it would be a bit thin, even in a culture which is increasingly moving towards a disturbingly new genetic determinism, as ours is. My credentials for being here this evening are more than genetic. I have worked for nearly 30 years as a sociologist centrally concerned with issues to do with health and the division of labour, especially the division of labour between men and women. Like most people's careers, my own was not the product of carefully considered rational choice. A crucial biographical moment – and I mention it only because it is germaine to the substance of my talk – occurred in 1969 when in the act of dusting my husband's bookshelves (he was a sociologist, too, so he had a lot of books) I picked up one on the sociology of work and noticed that housework was almost entirely missing from it. It appeared only as an aspect of the feminine role enabling women to be satisfied with low status poorly paid jobs outside the home; this allowed men to have the high status highly paid ones. Had my husband taught the sociology of health – which in those days was called medical sociology – I would probably have been equally disturbed to note that women's unpaid health care in the home was missing from that as well.

Gardens of Eden

In 1988 the Acheson report on the future of the public health function in

England talked fashionably about the 'intersectoral' nature of public health. The report quoted from the World Health Organization document on *Targets for Health for All* to the effect that 'the key to solving many health problems lies outside the health sector or is in the hands of the people themselves ...'[2] When we turn to the later (1992) *Health of the Nation* report, we find a section at the back entitled 'Key areas and the health of people in specific groups of the population'. The groups mentioned here are infants and children, elderly people, women, people from black and ethnic minorities, working class people, and people with disabilities, in that order.[3] In other words, middle aged, middle class white men are the dominant group, according to which the needs of other groups can be regarded as specific.

The theme of my lecture is the relation between these two points: the responsibility of the people for producing their own health, on the one hand, and the socially structured differences between men and women, on the other. It isn't, of course, fashionable these days to talk about gender: we are in what some people describe as the 'post-feminist' era. This means two things: either it means, we've solved all those problems to do with gender equality, or it means we're absolutely fed up with feminism and now is the time to move on to more important matters. But underlying my talk is the argument, which I might as well spell out now, that issues to do with the relative positions of men and women are absolutely critical to an understanding both of factors shaping the public health, and of the way ahead in terms of improving it. From this perspective, gender inequalities are as crucial as class inequality and inequalities between people of different ethnic groups. We live in a profoundly unequal society, but some people are more unequal than others. This inequality damages health. But it also *itself* proceeds from an unequal division of labour in health care work.

I want to try to link the gender division of labour in health care with two other themes: the first of these is the epidemiological evidence connecting socially supportive relationships with positive health outcomes; the second is the enduring puzzle of the division of labour in health itself: the fact that men die more while women seem to be sicker. In trying to accomplish these tasks, I shall draw rather cursorily on a wide range of publications and on three particular research projects carried out in my research unit in London. Two of these concern children and young people's attitudes to health,[4,5] while the third is a longitudinal study of social support and motherhood.[6]

The Matter With Eve

But I'll begin in a place you will all recognise: the Garden of Eden. The Irish writer George Bernard Shaw once wrote a play about the Garden of Eden called *Back to Methuselah*. In the first scene, Adam and Eve are in the Garden of Eden. Adam comes across a dead animal, and both he and Eve are disturbed by this reminder of death in the midst of life – that very substance and business of public health, of course. But Adam and Eve react differently to the reminder of mortality.

'You must be careful,' says Eve, the good housewife, to Adam, 'Promise me
you will be careful'.

Adam objects that there's little point in being careful, as something fatal is
bound to happen to him sooner or later. Then he realises with horror that the
same is true for his helpmate Eve. 'You must never put yourself in danger of
stumbling,' he instructs, 'You must not move about. You must sit still. I will
take care of you and bring you what you want.'

Eve's not over the moon about this idea that she should spend the rest of
her life sitting still and being dependent on Adam. In any case, she observes,
she really has no time to think about herself – she's kept far too busy thinking
about Adam. She has to think about Adam, because as she tells him in no
uncertain terms, 'You are lazy; you are dirty; you neglect yourself; you are
always dreaming; you would eat bad food and become disgusting if I did not
watch you and occupy myself with you'.[7]

Provision of health care and gender

Most of the world's primary health care is carried out by women. Women's
health care work is sometimes paid – as in the case of nurses, health visitors,
social workers, and other professions allied to medicine – or it is unpaid. In
the home, it is predominantly women who care for men and for children and
other dependents. These activities are commonly called housework, and the
people who do it are usually called housewives. These terms effectively disguise
the importance of the health work done in the home, but they also make an
important point in linking personal health work to public health concerns.
Caring for health is both about personal care – ensuring that people eat good
food, are kept warm and clean, and so forth – and about providing a health-
promoting material environment which facilitates the individual striving towards
good health. As the sociologist Hilary Graham has put it:

'Providing for health involves all the basic domestic activities we associate
with the maintenance of a home. It involves the provision of a materially secure
environment: warm, clean accommodation where both young and old can be
protected against danger and disease ... the purchase of food and the provision
of a diet sufficient in quantity and quality to meet their nutritional needs ...
the provision of a social environment conducive to normal health and development ... orchestrating social relations within the home ... to minimize
health-damaging insecurities'.[8]

'New Man' Failed to Reach Manhood
The point about social relations is an important one, to which I'll return later.
But first, I want to consider some of the ways in which this gender division of
labour manifests itself both within and outside the home. We have all heard
of the 'new man': the question is: does he really exist? Data on the domestic
division of labour in British households in 1984 and 1987 do not indicate that
things are moving fast in the direction of gender equality.[9] In a study of

adolescent health carried out in six London schools in 1990,[4] 15 and 16 year olds had already established a clear gender-differentiated pattern in responsbility for household tasks (fig 1). Note particularly the column entitled 'Making meals for others'. There was almost no difference between the frequency with which the young men and young women in this study made meals for themselves.

Gender and meanings of parenthood

	Mothers % (no)	Fathers % (no)
Employed full time (30 h or more)	53 (29)	94 (29)
Fits employment round family	98 (49)	43 (13)
Fits family round employment	34 (16)	74 (20)
Conflict between role as parent and individual fulfilment	44 (24)	41 (11)
Mothers and fathers are different	82 (44)	75 (21)
Main responsibility for young person:		
Mother	35 (19)	3 (1)
Father	0 (0)	10
Both	28 (15)	48 (14)
Negative feelings about young person leaving home	31 (16)	11 (3)
Worries a lot about young person	48 (26)	7 (2)
Influence over young person's activities:		
None	14 (6)	35 (8)
Some	63 (27)	39 (9)
A lot	23 (10)	26 (6)
Effect of young person on parental relationship:		
None	54 (27)	46 (13)
Positive	8 (4)	25 (7)
Negative/mixed	38 (19)	29 (8)
Effect of parental relationship on young person:		
None	38 (17)	42 (11)
Positive	7 (3)	31 (8)
Negative/mixed	56 (25)	27 (7)
Successful in bringing up teenager	60 (32)	69 (18)

Based on total of 55 mothers and 31 fathers; percentages are calculated on total numbers answering particular questions.

(Source: ref 4).

The table shows data from the same study[4] relating to the parents of the young people in question. Mothers, compared with fathers, are far more likely to fit their employment round the needs of their families. They are also much more likely to worry about their children. Like women's greater share of health care

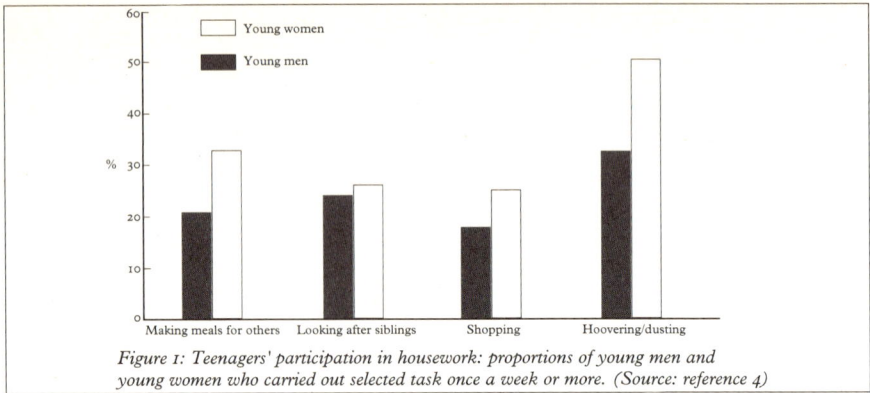

Figure 1: Teenagers' participation in housework: proportions of young men and young women who carried out selected task once a week or more. (Source: reference 4)

work, otherwise known as housework, their tendency to worry about health, like Eve in the Garden of Eden, starts young. As teenagers, girls are considerably more likely than boys to worry about health.[5]

Worries about health in young people

The next two questions are, what do teenagers worry about, and does worrying do them any good? Worries about health are bound up with the ways in which health is perceived. A crucial theme here is the extent to which health is seen as a matter of individual lifestyle or a product of environmental factors (or both). In one of our studies of young people and health we asked young children (9–10 year olds) to draw pictures of the factors in daily life they thought contributed to health and to illhealth.[1] Figure 2 shows a drawing by a 10 year old boy in an inner city school.

The healthy factors he drew included vitamins, weights, exercise machines, running and jogging, ambulances and hospitals, and healthy food. Another boy at the same school identified the following as unhealthy: sweets, smoking, fire, water (sometimes), tanks, car fumes, bombs, germs, factories, and John Major. The children's material environments affected their perceptions of health and illhealth, as can be seen from the drawing in fig 3 done by a girl in an urban school: moving from chips and drugs and chocolate and sweets and alcohol and pills to cars, suicide, diet, red meat, nuclear bombs, bedsits, police, stupid doctors and – yes – John Major again.

These drawings can be analyzed in many different ways, apart from the incidence of spelling mistakes. I am not here to talk about education but about health; however, at the risk of being unpopular among educationalists, I shall note that schools, teachers, and school dinners cropped up fairly often as bad for health. The identification of schools as health damaging environments is confirmed by other work which has looked at children's perspectives on health and education.[10] One interesting point which emerges from the children's drawings is the tendency for the health services to turn up as both good for health and bad for it. A second conclusion would reasonably be that these children have a fairly sophisticated knowledge of the common health education

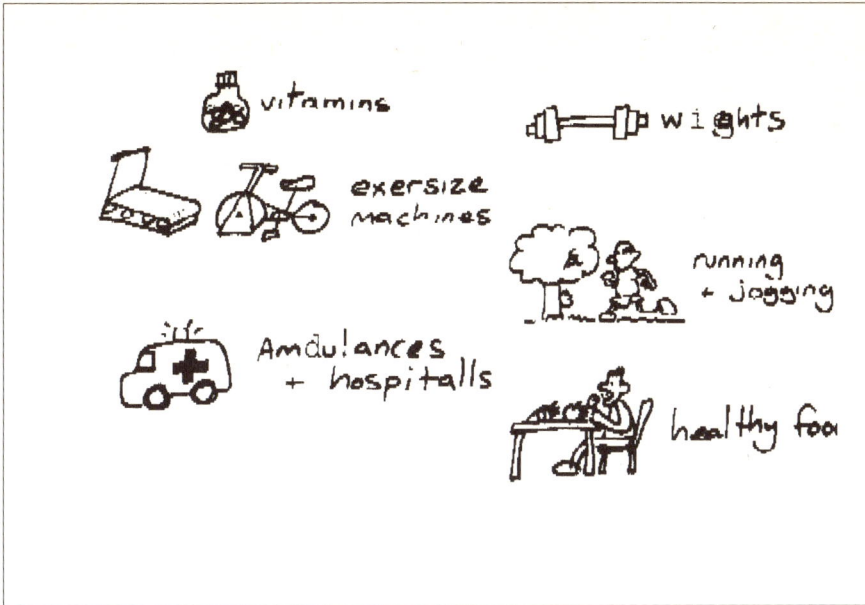

Figure 2: Childeren's beliefs about healthy factors in daily life: drawing by a 10 year old boy in an inner city school. (Source: reference 4.)

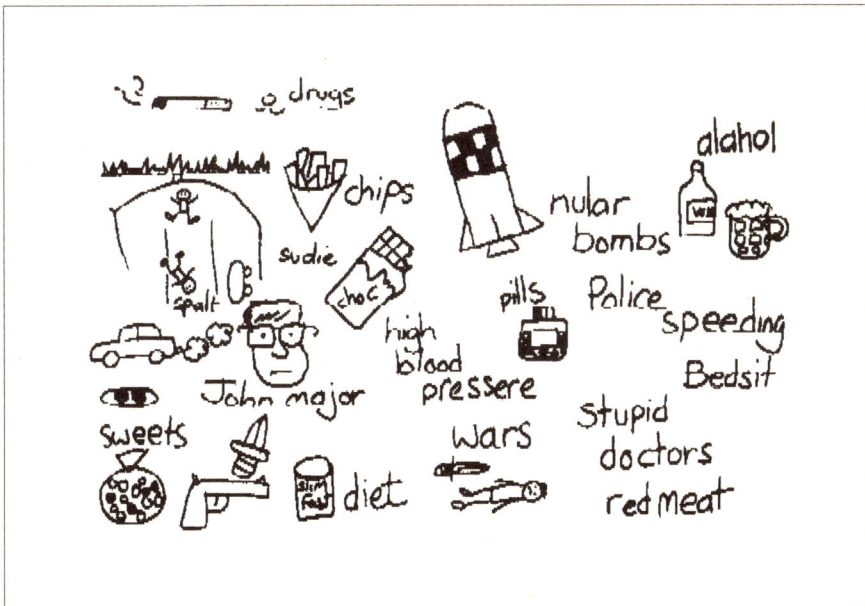

Figure 3: Childeren's beliefs about unhealthy factors in daily life: drawing by a 10 year old girl in an urban school. (Source: reference 4.)

messages. They know that a poor diet, drugs, smoking, and drinking are bad for health. They know that exercise and a good diet are good for health. But thirdly – and this is the conclusion I want to draw for the purposes of my talk this evening – what is notable is the lack of distinction in many of the drawings between individual lifestyle factors on the one hand, and material/environmental factors on the other. It is here, however, that we notice a gender difference: boys are more likely to focus on individual lifestyle factors and girls are more likely to combine these with aspects of the wider environment, from homelessness to nuclear war.

Other data from these two studies help to answer the question: what do men and women worry about? Young men are more likely to worry about unemployment, while young women go for AIDS, cancer, death, and nuclear war. These worries are related to health: more young women than young men think that AIDS will affect their future health; other important factors are what's happening to the ozone layer, the use of chemicals in food, and nuclear war. young men seem to be more concerned with traffic. When it comes to what teenagers consider to be the most important things in life, these are mainly job security and health for young men, whereas young women pick out happiness, a happy family, friends, and love.[4]

I want next to try to move on from all these 'soft' data to the 'harder' epidemiological concern about the links between socially supportive relationships on the one hand, and the broad picture of health and illness, on the other.

Friends for life?

In a study of Nazi concentration camp survivors, the people who had most problems recovering from their ordeal were those who were moved from camp to camp during the war; those who stayed in the same camp did better.[11] A study of mice showed that mice placed in a conflict situation were more likely to develop hypertension when with strange mice than with their litter mates.[12] Researchers looking at the growth of barley seeds demonstrated that seeds watered from a beaker which had been held for 15 minutes by a healer grew faster and taller than seeds watered with a more standard method.[13] In Alameda County, California, part of a State Health Department Human Population Laboratory study, people who lacked social and community ties were two to three times more likely to have died between initial data collection and a nine year follow up.[14] These disparate examples all come from the same body of literature, one which has burgeoned enormously over the last 20 years – the study of the links between social support and health. Lisa Berkman, the American epidemiologist who has specialised in this field, had this to say about it in a review published in 1984:

'From shopping bags in California bearing 'Friends make good medicine' to editorials in the *Journal of the American Medical Association*, 'A friend, Not an Apple a Day will Help Keep the Doctor Away', the message is that social support is both good preventive and curative medicine. Like chicken soup, its

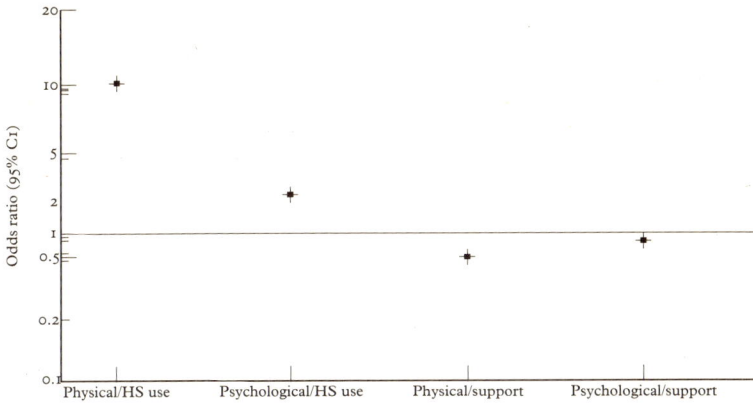

Figure 4: Association between health service (HS) use, social support, and physical and psychological health outcomes, adjusted for social class and previous health problems in mothers one year after giving birth. (Source: reference 23 by permission of Oxford University Press)

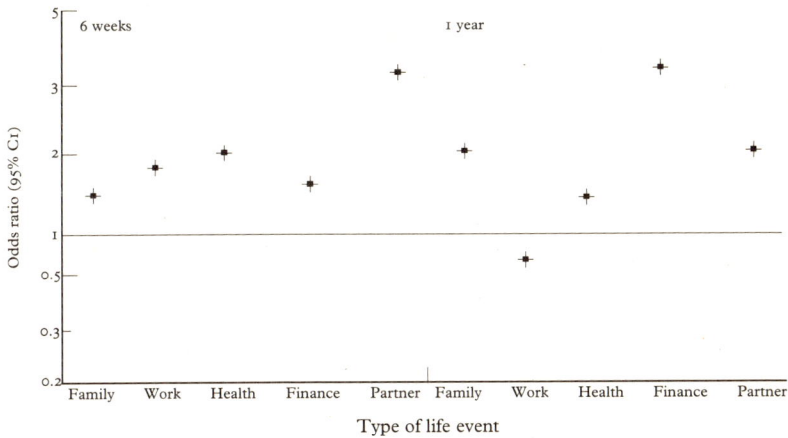

Figure 4: Association between psychological health and life events adjusted for social class and previous health outcomes in mothers six weeks and one year after giving birth.
(Source: reference 25 by permission of Oxford University Press)

powers are believed to be pervasive, the reasons for its effects are unknown, and knowledge of its qualities is widespread and based on folk wisdom ... From interactions among mice litter mates to collegiality among university graduates evidence has been garnered to support the notion that social ties are related to good health and well-being'.[15]

We now have good evidence that people who have close social relationships with other people have better physical and mental health.[16] The obvious rejoinder, that both good health and close social relationships are due to some other factor such as material advantage or better past health, does not explain this link. For example, in the Alameda Country Study, the relationship between lower mortality and high social support held independently of previous physical health status, social class, smoking, alcohol use, level of physical activity, obesity, ethnicity, life satisfaction and use of preventive health services.[14] A number of prospective studies show that the extent to which people are embedded in socially supportive relationships and networks is a strong predictor of health and morbidity, and of life *versus* death. Two examples of this link from the reproductive field are the well known work of Marshall Klaus and colleagues in the US showing the impact of social support in *labour* on health outcomes for mothers and babies,[17] and the findings from a controlled trial of social support during *pregnancy* I carried out with colleagues in 1985–9.[6] In this study, there was improvement in a range of health outcomes among women offered social support during pregnancy and their babies. These included both physical and psychosocial outcomes.

Never marry a man

The social support in both these cases was provided by women. There is a large body of evidence suggesting that social relationships with women are more health-promoting than social relationships with men.[18] Thus, marriage is generally better for men's than for women's health because men are married to women whereas women are married to men. Women generally benefit more from relationships with friends and relatives, which run predominantly along same-sex lines. When married men are asked in whom they confide, the answer is their wives, whereas married women asked the same question give a different answer: friends.[19] Research gives us some pointers as to why this should be so. For example, men tend to define intimacy as 'doing things together' whereas women tend to define it in terms of talking and listening.[20] Women disclose more than men do in close social relationships.[21] In surveys of help-seeking behaviour, women are more likely to be mentioned as helpers.[22]

Health services may not improve health

One of the research studies in which I've been involved recently is a re-analysis of data from our social support study as part of an Economic and Social Research Council (ESRC) initiative on what the council somewhat misleadingly terms 'personal welfare' (the renaming under Thatcher of the ESRC which used to be the *Social Science* Research Council was accompanied by the banning

of unfashionable terminology to do with public or more social forms of welfare).
In this re-analysis we have attempted to quantify the effects of different types
of social support on health, and to compare the role of social support with the
role of the health services. On reflection, this was a pretty silly thing to try to
do, as it was bound to take us into sticky and even more unfashionable waters.
It did. What we found is summarised in fig 4:[23] a tendency for social support
to improve health and for health service use to have the opposite effect. I have
no doubt that the highlighting of health service use as not automatically health-
promoting may be regarded as controversial. We were somewhat surprised by
it ourselves. However, when you place it in the context of the health needs of
this particular population (pregnant women and mothers of young children),
and view it in the light of what we already know about user satisfaction in these
groups, it ceases to be so surprising. The common complaints of lack of
continuity of care, long waiting times, and other practical difficulties, and 'ritual'
medical encounters with unsympathetic health professionals hardly add up to
a recipe for health.[24] The relevance of the health services to the promotion of
the public health is the fundamental question here.

Going back to the analysis of the social support and pregnancy study date,
when we looked at where the social support came from, the three sources most
related to health outcomes were the women's own mothers, their friends, and
the research midwife. Figure 5 shows the relationships between different types
of life events and women's psychological health six weeks and one year after
childbirth.[25] Again, we have controlled for previous health problems and or
social class. Most types of life event have a negative effect on women's health.
At six weeks, the category of life events most strongly related to the mothers'
psychological health was associated either with the relationship with the partner
or with events in his life. For example, women who had problems with their
partners were three times more likely to have poor rather than good psychological
health.

Does caring for health do women any good?

Differences between men and women in mortality and morbidity exist in all
developed countries. It's a familiar pattern: women have lower death rates than
men at virtually every age and for most causes of death. But despite this
advantage in mortality, they have higher rates of non-fatal acute and chronic
conditions, and experience more illness diversity than men: they also have higher
rates of service use.[26] The sex difference is especially marked for indices of
mental well-being. It is a consistent finding of epidemiological research that
women experience higher rates of psychological distress and depression than
men.[27] Various explanations have been offered for this female specialisation in
poor quality of life: the three main ones are (1) that it's women's biology that
makes them ill, (2) that it's their social roles, and (3) that they aren't really ill
at all, they're only inventing it.

While there is little evidence for the first hypothesis, there is a good deal in

favour of the second. Poor emotional well-being in married women compared
with other gender and marital states, for example, emerges as a consistent
finding in much of the literature.[28] The sex difference is heightened when
non-employed married women are compared with all other categories.

The 'artefactual' explanation – that women make up their symptoms – is an
interesting one, and this is not the place to discuss it in detail. We live in a
culture with a long tradition of discounting women's experiences as unimportant.
Unsurprisingly, this is reflected in strategies for researching health. For example,
tiredness or fatigue, a symptom much more frequently reported by women than
by men, is conceptualised in much of the research literature as a *psychological*
rather than a *physical* symptom. If you redefine it as a physical symptom, then
women's health is worse than men's controlling for social class, household
income, marital status, and relationship to paid work.[29] What this analysis
suggests is that it is women's worse physical health that leads to the gender
differences in mental health, and not the other way around; women *feel* sick
because they *are* sick.

An interesting analysis by Lois Verbrugge, who has been much occupied
professionally by the puzzle of these gender differences, shows that the strongest
risk factors for poor health status are also those which show the greatest gender
differences.[30] This analysis, which used data from a large study carried out in
Detroit, also showed that if these risk factors (which included such items as
non-employment, role stress, and low mastery) are controlled for, the overall
differences in morbidity by gender are substantially narrowed.

Physical work and caring as factors in poorer health
There are two gender differences in daily life that underlie this finding of
women's poorer health. One is the physical burden of work associated with
women's domestic roles, and the other is the physical and psychological costs
to women of being the ones who care. A re-analysis of General Household
Survey data shows relationships between the extent of the domestic work-load
and the reporting of physical symptoms.[31] This is perhaps another indicator of
the importance of research in establishing the strength of common sense:
working hard makes you tired and may damage your health in other ways.
Another aspect of our cultural tradition which influences the way we concep-
tualise health and its links with the physical and social environment is our focus
on the health hazards of work outside the home. In trying to understand what
makes people sick we ignore the conditions of their domestic lives; yet it is
these very conditions that form the physical context for much of women's
primary health care work. Working conditions in the home may be more
dangerous than those in the public domain.[32] The Italian social scientist Patrizia
Romito has shown how the hazards of women's domestic roles are systematically
ignored in the literature and medical practices relating to risk and pregnancy
outcome. Full time housewives have worse pregnancy outcomes than women
employed outside the home, controlling for the 'healthy worker' effect.

Risks associated with 'women's' work
Romito also demonstrates that the conditions of women's work more generally pose important risks that are often not taken into account. For example, one traditional feminine activity is that of nursing. Nurses have high rates of preterm and low birthweight babies, and their work involves them in tasks whose links with these outcomes are well known: standing for long periods, lifting and moving heavy loads, the strain of night shift. Moreover, nurses, like anaesthetists and radiologists – also predominantly female occupations – are exposed to directly teratogenic risks. 'Protective' labour legislation can control these hazards to some extent. But a double standard operates. For example, women in the United States are not allowed to work in industries involving contact with lead, but the exclusion is limited to heavy industries where salaries are relatively high. Women are not excluded from light industrial work involving lead such as ceramics where salaries are much lower, and a higher proportion of the workers are women.[33]

Living conditions and health
The ways in which working and living circumstances damage health have, of course, been known for many years. Whenever parents of young children are interviewed about their child health work, for instance, the significance of physical features of the home and its environment emerge as absolutely crucial. In a study conducted by Berry Mayall in London several years ago in which mothers of under 3s were interviewed about how they kept their children healthy, a third of working class mothers identified aspects of housing they were powerless to alter (such as badly placed doors in rented property, steep stairs, and non-childproof windows) as major dangers to their children's health.[34] Parental concerns about the links between damp housing and respiratory illness in children prompted a survey in Glasgow which did, indeed, establish a connection.[35]

Poverty and its impact on health represent another unfashionable subject. Here the links between class and gender inequalities are close: widening class inequalities in health are associated with increasing gender differences, as demographic trends establish women and children as the single largest and fastest growing poverty group.[36] This means that a growing proportion of women's health care work in the home is accomplished in conditions of poverty. I want to say a little bit about caring in conditions of material constraint before trying to bring all the various themes I've mentioned together in the form of conclusions about agendas for public health work.

Cigarettes – the stressed carer's friends
One of the things women do when they're trying to look after other people in difficult circumstances is that they smoke. Smoking is increasingly a marker for poverty, and it is increasingly women, and not men, who are taking up and continuing the smoking habit.[37]

There is no evidence that women smoke out of ignorance about its health effects. On the contrary, most are sharply aware that smoking is bad for them. The point is that their smoking is 'good' for the people they have to look after – young children, difficult adolescents, demanding husbands, elderly relatives. Smoking provides a strategy for calming the nerves and coping with stress, a fact that is sometimes literally expressed in the metaphor of the smoke ring: the young overburdened socially disadvantaged mother of two or three children securing a break from her maternal work by sitting down, having a cigarette, and retiring for a moment to the world inside the smoke ring where she can find enough energy to carry on.[38] Women's smoking is intimately related to social deprivation, stress, and disadvantage.[39] As one mother in our social support study said:[6]

'I tried to give up, but I get so as I want to kill everybody. I don't think it's worth it at the moment ... at the hospital, they have asked me again if I smoke ... The doctor at the clinic, he said I really should give it up. He was the same doctor I had last time. I felt so sorry for him. I couldn't give up. I told him I would cut down ... If I'd gone back and he'd said, 'Have you?' I would have said, 'Yes' ... you don't want to hurt their feelings, do you?'

Note this woman's sensitivity to the doctor's feelings. Being aware of other people's feelings may mean that you give them inaccurate information: this has implications for the research base of public health. In this study we compared the information about smoking rates provided by the same women to health professionals in hospital, to researchers in an interview, and in a postal questionnaire, and found the highest smoking rates reported in the postal questionnaire.[40]

Gender, social relations, and the public health

There is nothing biologically inevitable about the gender differences I've been discussing. All the evidence is that these result from an unequal pattern of socialisation in which girls are sensitised to the need to care for others and boys are given the message that real men don't care.[41] Real men also don't do housework, and studies of gender differences among children and adults in household work show that women do most, followed by girls, followed by boys, followed by men.[42] We live in a culture which holds up certain images of family life and of femininity and masculinity as ideal; yet there is much weighty evidence showing the strains these ideal formulas impose.[43]

So to sum all this up: the first point is a conceptual one. In carrying the cultural division between the private and public domains – the world of the home and the world outside it – into the field of health, those whose professional concerns are with researching or promoting health are committing a basic error. Health care work isn't only done by those who are paid to do it – doctors, nurses, health visitors, health educators. Most of it is done by people who aren't paid at all. This health care division of labour is fundamental to the public health. Underlying what we might call invisible health care work is a different and more accurate model of how health is 'really' produced: one which combines caring – social support in technical language – and the more usual physical-technical strategies.

The Importance of caring

Thus, a second point concerns the best way to promote health. Health is most effectively promoted in the context of caring relationships. It is when people feel cared for and cared about that they are most likely to feel well. There is an important lesson here for the health services. Historically speaking, the evolution of high technology services has been at the cost of caring services. It is not impossible for a health care system to provide high technology care in a caring way, but this will only happen when the provision of *care* in the generic sense is recognised to be a legitimate and primary goal shaping the form the health services take. This means that an important task ahead for those concerned with the public health is a radical look at what health services actually achieve, beyond the rhetoric which equates them automatically with health promotion. As Jane Lewis has shown in her history of the development of community medicine,[44] public health medicine became progressively alienated from its wider environmental function in the UK from the late 1940s on. Public health gain came to be equated increasingly with counts of service provision – numbers of hospital beds provided, of children inspected. Under the new NHS in 1993 there is a real impetus to re-evaluate the role of the health services, though driven by economic cost-cutting motives rather than by a rational philosophy of health promotion. It will be essential in future to ensure that economic costs and benefits are not the only criteria used in reshaping services for health, and that these do not develop so as to inflate the health-damaging gender divisions I've talked about.

Towards equality

Thirdly, one important means of improving the public health would be to dissolve the socially imposed differences between the life-chances of men and women. Specifically, the same need as was expressed in the early 1900s and the early 1970s (the two most recent periods of feminist activity) to improve the social and economic position of women still holds. Housework, well paid employment work, caring, and poverty ought to be more equally distributed between the sexes than they are now.

Educating the health care educators

Fourthly, much of the rhetoric today is about educating people about health in order to lessen the burden on the health services of morbidity due to unhealthy lifestyles. Women are the prime targets of these health education messages. I would suggest on the basis of the evidence I've presented to you that the health education message ought to be the other way around: it is the health educators who need educating about what women as primary health workers themselves know about health. The broader point here is one about the importance of daily, lifelong experience and the knowledge derived from this in contrast to the professionalised agendas of the various groups of experts we have put in charge of life in modern industrialised societies. Some years ago, the science fiction writer Ursula LeGuin wrote a short essay called *The Space Crone*. In this she considers what might happen when a space ship arrives from some other planet and the captain says there is room for one passenger from earth, a passenger who can convey to the natives of his own planet the essence of the experience of life on earth. 'I suppose,' says LeGuin, 'what most people would want to do is provide them with a fine, bright, brave young man, highly educated and in peak physical condition. A Russian cosmonaut would be ideal (American astronauts are mostly too old). There would surely be hundreds, thousands of volunteers ... But I would not pick any of them ...' says LeGuin:

> What I would do is go down to the local Woolworth's, or the local village marketplace, and pick an old woman, over sixty ... Her hair would not be red or blonde or lustrous dark, her skin would not be dewy fresh, she would not have the secret of eternal youth ... She has worked hard at small, unimportant jobs all her life, jobs like cooking, cleaning, bringing up kids... The trouble is, she will be very reluctant to volunteer ... 'You ought to send one of those scientist men ... Maybe Dr Kissinger should go?' ... 'Me?' she'll say, just a trifle slyly, 'But I never did anything' ...

But it won't wash. She knows though she won't admit it, that Dr Kissinger has not gone and will never go where she has gone, that the scientists ... have not done what she has done. Into the space ship, Granny".[45]

References

1. Oakley, A. Eugenics, social medicine and the career of Richard Titmuss in Britain 1935–1950. *British Journal of Sociology* 1991; 42(2):165–94.
2. *Public health in England: The report of the committee of inquiry into the future development of the public health function*. London: HMSO, 1988:9.
3. The Secretary of State for Health. *The health of the nation: A strategy for health in England*. London: HMSO, 1992.
4. Brannen J, Dodd K, Oakley A, Storey P. *Young people, health and family life*. Milton Keynes: Open University Press, 1994.
5. Bendelow G, Oakley A. *Children and young people's beliefs about cancer*. London: Social Science Research Unit, 1993.
6. Oakley A. *Social support and motherhood: The natural history of a research project*. Oxford: Basil Blackwell, 1992.
7. Shaw GB. *The complete plays of Bernard Shaw*. London: Odhams Press, 1934.
8. Graham H. *Women, health and the family*. Brighton, Sussex: Harvester, 1984.
9. Jowell R, Witherspoon S, Brook L. *British Social Attitudes: the 5th report*. London: Gower, 1988.
10. Mayall B. Keeping healthy at home and at school: 'it's my body so it's my job'. *Sociology of Health and Illness* 1993; 15:469–871.
11. Davidson S. Massive psychic traumatization and social support. *Journal of Psychosomatic Research* 1979; 23:395–402.

12. Henry J, Meehan J, Stephens P. The use of psychosocial stimuli to induce prolonged hypertension in mice. *Psychosomatic Medicine* 1967;29:408.

13. Grad B. A telekinetic effect on plant growth. *International Journal of Parapsychology* 1963;5:117–33.

14. Berkman LF, Syme L. Social networks, host resistance, and mortality: a nine-year follow-up study of Alameda County residents. *Am J Epidemiol* 1979;109(2):186–204.

15. Berkman LF. Assessing the physical health effects of social networks and social support. *Am Rev Public Health* 1984; 5:413–32.

16. Cohen S, Syme L, eds. *Social support and health.* New York: Academic Press, 1985.

17. Klaus MH, Kennell JJ, Robertson SS, Sosa R. Effects of social support during parturition on maternal and infant morbidity. *BMJ* 1986;6:585–7.

18. Belle D. The stress of caring: women as providers of social support. In: Goldberger L, Breznitz S, eds. *Handbook of stress: theoretical and clinical aspects.* New York: The Free Press, 1982.

19. Lowental M, Hanen C. Interaction and adaptation: intimacy as a critical variable. *American Sociological Review* 1968;33:390–400.

20. Helgerson VS, Shaver PR, Dyer M. Prototypes of intimacy and distance in same-sex and opposite-sex relationships. *Journal of Social and Personal Relationships* 1987;4195–233.

21. Duck S. *Friends, for life: the psychology of personal relationships.* Hemel Hempstead, Hertfordshire: Harvester Wheatsheaf, 1991.

22. Kessler R. Social factors in psychopathology: stress, social support and coping processes. *Am Rev Psychol* 1985;36:531–72.

23. Oakley A, Rigby AS, Hickey D. Love or money: social support, class inequality and health of women and children. *European Journal of Public Health* 1994 (in press).

24. Scott-Samuel A. Why don't they want our health services? *Lancet* 1980;23:412–13.

25. Oakley A, Rigby AS, Hickey D. *Life stress, support and class inequality: explaining the health of women and children. European Journal of Public Health* 1994;4:81–91.

26. Wingard DL. The sex differentials in morbidity, mortality and life style. In: Breslow L, Fielding JE, Lave LB eds. *Annual review of public health.* 1984;5:433–58. Palo Alto, California: Annual Reviews.

27. Pugliesi K. Women and mental health: Two traditions of feminist research. *Women and Health* 1992;19(2/3):43–68.

28. Gove WS, Tudor JF. Adult sex roles and mental illness. *American Journal of Sociology* 1973;178:50–73.

29. Popay J, Bartley M, Owen C. Gender inequalities in health: social position, affective disorders and minor physical morbidity. *Soc Sci Med* 1993;36(1):21–32.

30. Verbrugge L. Unveiling higher morbidity for men: the story. In: Riley MW ed. *Social structures and human lives.* Newbury Park: Sage Publications, 1988.

31. Bartley M, Popay J, Plewis I. *Domestic work-load, paid employment and women's experiences of ill-health.* London: Thomas Coram Research Unit, 1991.

32. Kowarzik U, Popay J. *That's women's work: report on women's unpaid labour in the home.* London: London Research Centre, 1989.

33. Romito P, Hovelaque F. Changing approaches in women's health: new insights

and new pitfalls in prenatal preventive care. *International Journal of Health Services* 1987;17(2):241–58.

34. Mayall B. *Keeping children healthy*. London: Allen and Unwin, 1986.

35. Martin CJ, Platt SD, Hunt SM. Housing conditions and ill-health. *BMJ* 1987;294:1125–7.

36. Thomas Coram Research Unit/University of Warwick. *Women and poverty: exploring the research and policy agenda*. London: Thomas Coram Research Unit, 1989.

37. Graham H. Women's smoking and family health. *Soc Sci Med* 1987;25:47–56.

38. Graham H. Smoking in pregnancy: the attitudes of expectant mothers. *Soc Sci Med* 1976;10:399–405.

39. Oakley A. Smoking in pregnancy: smokescreen or risk factor? Towards a materialist analysis. *Sociology of Health and Illness* 1989;11(4):311–35.

40. Oakley A., Rajan L., Robertson P. A comparison of different sources of information on pregnancy and childbirth. *Journal of Biosocial Science* 1990;27:477–87.

41. Chodorow N. *The reproduction of mothering: psychoanalysis and the sociology of gender*. Berkeley, California: University of California Press, 1978.

42. Frones I, Jensen A, Solberg A. National report for Norway. *Childhood as a social phenomenon project*. Vienna: European Centre for Social Welfare Policy and Research, 1992.

43. Oakley A. Conventional families. In: Rapoport RN, Rapoport R, Fogarty MP. *Families in Britain*. London: Routledge and Kegan Paul, 1982.

44. Lewis J. *What price community medicine?* Brighton, Sussex: Wheatsheaf Books, 1986.

45. LeGuin U. The space crone. In: *Dancing at the edge of the world*. New York: Harper and Row, 1990.

Public participation in health care quality

Duncan memorial lecture. Lowell S Levin. Department of Epidemiology and Public Health, Division of International Health, Yale University School of Medicine, 60 College Street, PO Box 3333, New Haven, Connecticut 06510–8034, USA. Presented at the University of Liverpool. 7 December 1994.

With my presentation there will have been an even dozen Duncan lecturers. It is extraordinary how the work and character of William Henry Duncan has caused the selection of such a diverse array of themes. Each of the Duncan lectures, however, found in Dr Duncan's work a strand of common cause with their own interests. And I am no exception. Duncan knew from his experience with the authorities, be they governmental or professional, that for public health to advance it must build a public constituency of informed citizens. The horrendous poverty of Liverpool, its crowded housing and lack of sanitation were, of course, obvious to the middle class but the powerful link of such conditions with high levels of morbidity and mortality needed Dr Duncan's documentation to build the basis for public understanding of the public health prevention option. This may have been the first time that a purposeful effort was made to enlist public support for a specific public health action.

Since Duncan's day, of course, there has been a steady increase in the encouragement of public participation in moving the public health agenda forward. Progress toward full public participation has not, however, been constant or without professional/governmental resistance. Sharon Arnstein, an American citizen health advocate, developed nearly 25 years ago the so called 'ladder of participation' that described eight levels of participation. These started with informing, consultation, and placation and moved to three degrees of what Arnstein referred to as 'citizen power' – partnership, delegated power, and citizen control.[1] Clearly Dr Duncan climbed the first several steps on the ladder and was probably inclined to seek public-professional partnership as well. But nearly a century had passed before serious strategic consideration was given to involving the public as partners in health planning, delegating specific power of self determination in health care, or placing citizens in full control of the health enterprise.

We are presently a long way from the latter and are still tentative about 'partnership' and lay self determination in health. We in the health and related professions remain quite caught up in the exclusivity of our 'qualifications' in health matters and view with suspicion the ability of ordinary citizens to provide criticism or even to comprehend the complexities of health actions, be they at the political or personal level. We are, at the same time, absolutely convinced of the scientific merit and wisdom of our professional expertise. Ordinary citizens have *beliefs* – we have *knowledge*. This, despite mounting evidence of public competence in health decision-making[2] concurrent with mounting evidence of the fallibility of the medical and public health professions.[3]

Of course, these two realities are not usually juxtaposed, but professional critiques of the lay role in health have an undercurrent of defensiveness. The view is that the proponents of the lay role, especially in personal care, are reacting critically to limitations of professional care.[4] Perhaps. But what this points out is the discomfort health professionals feel as they see the erosion of their power as health and health care become increasingly social ideas where many voices and many resources want to have their contributions acknowledged.

The popularisation of health does take its toll on traditional roles, traditional constructions of reality, and the egos invested in them. Is nothing sacred anymore, some ask? Does democratisation know no bounds? Will the time come when plebiscites will replace scientific inquiry to determine truth? Will citizen control, ending professional dominance,[5] as we have grown to know and cherish it, destroy health gains already achieved? Or are we entering a new era of health development where lay and professional collaboration, with full professional *and* public oversight will bring us closer to the World Health Organization's idealistic goal of health for all? What is going on here and where might it take us.

In my time with you this evening, I want to respond to these questions as they redefine health as common property, in its achievement, maintenance, and restoration. I cannot profess an unbiased view of consumerism and health, because I could not get away with it for very long anyway. Too many of my British colleagues in the College of Health and the Patients' Association have shared panels or podia with me as we challenged what in earlier days we called the establishment. What saves you (us) from my bias now is that I no longer have to rely on impressions, anecdotes, and rhetoric.

Lay initiatives in personal health care

Since the late 1970s there has been an extraordinarily productive research effort, largely in the UK, USA, and Canada that documents the extent and quality of lay initiatives in personal health care, social care, and most recently in the heretofore sacred domain of quality assurance. This is not to say that we have reached the promised land of a full text on how any, much less all, aspects of lay health actions perform, but the research agenda now clearly specifies the work yet to be done. We have a map and now we have the financial support of government who were previously reluctant to invest in an area of study some felt was antiestablishment. After all, some argued, if levels of self care are shown to be high, will this not be an indication that government services have failed to meet needs? Or, as some third world observers cautioned, promoting lay self care may be a 'sinister' plot to avoid government responsibility."[6]

Undoubtedly, some people in the industrialised countries feel the same way.[7] In this country, it was Dr John Fry who in effect said 'nonsense' to all of the above; self care is the base of the health care pyramid and essential for the efficacy of the overall health care system.[8] A decade later John Last in his classic study of self care practices forced consideration of lay practices in 'completing the clinical picture in general practice'.[9] Research began to build which documented the extent (Williamson and Danaher,[10] Pratt,[11] Freer,[12] Elliot-Binns,[13] Alpert, et al[14]) and efficacy of lay self care practices (Zapka,[15] Knapp and Knapp,[16] Litman,[17] Katz[18]).

Self care – a threat to the status quo

In 1975, what turned out to be a landmark or at least benchmark international symposium on the 'Role of the Individual in Primary Health Care', sponsored jointly by the University of Copenhagen and the University of California, Los Angeles was held in Copenhagen at the European headquarters of the World Health Organization. The symposium took a hard look at lay health care practices, clarified roles and functions, drew attention to relevant technical and social issues, and identified priority research needs. But acceptance of the lay contribution to health and especially to medical care was a tough struggle. Nothing came easy.

Indeed in my country, the government undertook a study of lay medical care practices which concluded that such practices represented 'rampant empiricism', antithetical to the health and welfare of the American people.[19] Never mind that 80 to 95% of *all* illness episodes were self cared for (and safely!). Never mind that 15 million people in the USA were in a given census year members of mutual aid groups. Twenty years ago my government, with the advice of health care authorities it is assumed, was seeking ways of stamping out the unauthorised practice of medicine albeit self directed within the family. Those who proposed expanding lay self care practices were viewed negatively by authorities, both governmental (regulatory) and professional (organised medicine). They were seen as promoting an 'empowerment strategy', a serious threat to the status quo. And indeed it was.

The women's health movement challenged medical authority in the boldest and most courageous of ways. Some women's clinics and education centres were shut down and their personnel jailed for allegedly practising medicine without a license. These women were saying 'enough!' to what they perceived as abuses in the professional medical treatment they received. They dared to 'go public' about these abuses and arm women with the knowledge and skills to take charge of their own bodies. The do it yourself vaginal examination using a speculum became the symbol of their struggle.

Self protection

In America, it was the women's health movement, and in particular The Women's Health Book Collective in Boston,[20] that first broadened the definition of self care to include concern for, and ways to protect oneself from, the hazards of professional medical services. Starkly put, women are seen by some health professionals as a disease. Many normal physiological phenomena are converted to pathologies, from puberty to birthing to menopause. Women are 'exposed' to medical care five to six times as much as are men. In the USA and Canada, nearly 60% of women will not reach their 65th birthday with an intact uterus! Caesarean section rates hover around 25%. Mammography screening fails to meet known epidemiological criteria for use. Ultrasound is excessively used in pregnancy. And women are overdosed with unnecessary regimen of prescribed medications. One Canadian physician summed it up:

> 'Over the last 16 years of medical practice, I have seen many women suffer needlessly because their doctors did not really listen to them, told them that physically based complaints were all in their heads and treated normal events in a women's life as if they were diseases. Time and again I have seen women paying a heavy price for the careless prescription of antibiotics, birth control pills, hormones, and tranquilizers.'[21]

In the United States, the relatively benign self care consumer movement began to reflect a concern for the quality of professional medical care and the personal skills required to be more self protecting. The challenges to the hegemony of medical professionals began to spread in the mid-70s beyond the borders of women's groups. A major rise in public awareness of the hazard of medical care came through the 1975 publication of Ivan Illich's severe critique of medicine as a source of multiple levels of iatrogenic complications. Many of you can recall the furore this little volume created in medical circles. Illich's work and his persona became an irresistible irritant. He hit a sensitive spot and opened public debate on a previously taboo topic: the fallibility of medicine. Who was this priest who dared to expose the secrets of priests of another calling? As a learned philosopher with international standing, Illich could not be dismissed lightly. Perversely, the health professionals could not get enough of him. Time and again he was asked to explain his position at conferences and seminars of medical practitioners and academics. His views began, as well, to attract the attention of lay voluntary health groups. He broadened awareness of the limits and hazards of medical care at physical, psychological, and socio-political levels.

End of the age of innocence

The age of public innocence regarding medical care and its supporting institutions was coming to a close in America. Soon a plethora of books on medicine's shortcomings began to make their way into the popular trade market. The most successful in the USA was Dr Robert S Mendelsohn's *Confessions of a Medical*

Heretic in which the author" ... tells you how to guard yourself against the harmful impact upon your life of doctors, drugs and hospitals."[22] A respected clinician, Mendelsohn was also chairman of the Medical Licensing Committee for the State of Illinois and a faculty member of the University of Illinois School of Medicine. His public testimony was a shock to the medical community. Some colleagues labelled him more a traitor than heretic. But public interest was keen, quickly making *Confessions* a best seller.

That same year (1979) Dr Richard Taylor, a member of the Doctors' Reform Society in Australia, wrote an equally audacious book, but a nonetheless meticulously documented account of the adverse effects of medical care. His book, *Medicine Out of Control*, had as its subtitle 'the Anatomy of a Malignant Technology'.[23] Now, Australians are a kind and gentle people not ordinarily given to hyperbole, much less to frontal attacks on respected social institutions. But Taylor's critique seems to have struck a responsive chord even among some general practitioners who had reservations about medical specialists who they charged did not encourage patients to make informed decisions regarding the appropriateness and safety of high tech medical procedures.

Another publicly oriented trade book, this time by an Australian lawyer and journalist, concentrated its attack not only on the 'huge hidden toll of medical malpractice in Australia, but also how the law enabled negligent and incompetent doctors to escape penalty ... [and] how medical defence organisations use an array of 'dirty tricks' to stifle legal action by patients.'[24] Arguably biased as a lawyer, author Stephen Rice does seem to have done a careful job of documentation as if preparing a legal brief. His work tapped another aspect of public concern about the quality of care issues: the belief that the medical establishment is an impenetrable club with little possibility for ordinary citizens to gain access to performance data on practitioners or institutional care. Such restricted access to quality of care information diminishes patients' capacity to make personal care decisions as well as sound political judgements about medical care reform. With regard to patient access to information, one contributor to the Victorian (Australia) Law Reform Commission's report on *Informed Decisions about Medical Procedures* wrote:

> Other doctors, however, still cling to the notion that 'doctor knows best'! They believe that their patients expect the doctor to tell them what to do, rather than to encourage them to make their own informed decisions. Confronted by this attitude, patients are often confused; they do not know what information they should be given, how to ask for it, or what they should do if they think that they have not been properly informed or suitably treated.[25]

Nor has the public been well informed about the efficacy of the medical care system. Even in medical care systems considered exemplary, such as Canada's, the overuse and sometimes misuse of high tech procedures is commonplace. Canadians are just now becoming aware of the reason for long waits for elective surgery, long emergency room queues and other apparent discrepancies between the image of having the best system and the reality of a 'rationed' service.[26]

Quality of medical care

Now, in order to make clear the basis for the growing public concern for the quality of medical care, I offer some aspects of the American experience. Iatrogenic complications are not frivolous matters there. The table shows a few examples which will give some sense of the magnitude of the problem.[27]

I do not mean to suggest that American medical care or medical care in other industrialised countries is a disaster. But we cannot ignore that old aphorism: one third of medical encounters help one third make things worse, and one third neither help or hurt.

Studies of the quality of medical care in the United States over the past 15 years, however, have shown no appreciable improvement in key indicators such as rates of nosocomial infection, medication errors, anaesthesia errors, unnecessary surgery (except the slight drop in caesarean sections), laboratory errors, and *x* ray diagnostic errors. With accelerated use of technology there is further room for complications at the hands of inadequately trained or supervised operators, as in the case of laparoscopic surgery.[29]

Current strategies for quality control have not obviously improved the situation. The combined efforts of hospital infections committees, surgical and medical audits, quality assurance review boards, and medical licensing boards does not seem to have contributed to a significant gradient of improvement. Even a new USA government oversight programme that attempts to track the movement of incompetent health care providers has not been sufficient. Similarly, the USA system for reporting defective hospital equipment has had little effect on the use of such equipment. Government hospital accrediting agencies do review, inspect, and approve hospitals, but 'in reality these organizations labor under inconsistent standards and yield poor inspection results .... missing two out of three quality-of-care problems related to physicians' care in hospitals.'[30] So it was inevitable that the public would perceive that its health interests were not being adequately protected by the government and professional agencies and that public pressure for reform was necessary.

The quality of medical care – some aspects of the US experience

- Only 10 to 20% of all procedures currently used in medical practice have been shown to be efficacious in controlled trial (OTA 1978).
- The reporting of a procedure's overuse or obsolescence has a very slow impact on the practice of medicine (Rand Corporation/UCLA 1987).
- Nearly a quarter of all hospital admission and 15% of doctors' office visits are unnecessary; and 53% of time spent in the hospital is medically unnecessary
- Five–10% of American physicians are incompetent to practise medicine, not including those with incapacities such as drug abuse, alcoholism.

- Laboratory testing: approximately two thirds of tests are useless to irrelevant, with an overall 4% error rate. In 1985 this error rate represented 140 million test results.

- Approximately 5% of patients in hospital, according to a 1984 Harvard study 'sustained injuries that resulted from their medical care and not the underlying disease'. 1.35% was ascribed to medical negligence.[28] This study, however, did not include a wide variety of treatment related injuries such as nosocomial infections, diagnostic errors, or unnecessary surgeries or unnecessary invasive testing.

- The nosocomial infection rate is now 5–10% of hospitalised patients.

- The medication (hospital) error rate *not* using a unit-dose system averages 11.6% of medication administrations.

- Five million surgical procedures are unnecessary (21% caesarean section rate).

- Twenty two per cent of hysterectomies are unnecessary (mostly involving women under 40 years).

Lay health care is increasing

At the same time, the strong base of public interest in personal health action in the US keeps growing. Now there is increased access to the technologies of medical care (note the 10 billion dollar do it yourself medical equipment industry), greater access to effective medication (switch from prescribed to over the counter products), and above all a tremendous acceleration in health and medical information via books and magazines, electronic media (12 TV doctors), and syndicated health columns in the daily press. One estimate is that there are over 7000 book titles in the general category of do it yourself medical care. The range of subjects runs from standard protocols text,[31] dealing with common medical problems,[32, 33] selecting appropriate medications,[34] to a plethora of holistic and alternative medical texts.[35] There is also a modest literature on self protection in medical care, although its appeal is largely confined to a rather sophisticated audience. One of the earliest of these texts was written by a physician who was seeking to encourage a new kind of patient '...assertive, questioning, capable of making decisions that are vital to his survival.'[36] The latest book, *When your Doctor Doesn't Know Best*, is subtitled '229 Errors Even the Best Doctors Make and How to Protect Yourself'.[37]

The People's Medical Society

America is arguably the world's most consumerist and litigious society. Americans have a core mistrust of government and professional associations devoted to the well being of their profession. And, as noted earlier, the reverse is true as well. American government agencies and health professional organisations, with few exceptions, were never keen on public empowerment in health. Professionals seem to hold all the cards. They are organised and, well financed, and influential with government authorities. The public, on the other hand, while increasingly better informed about health and medical care had no focal point for their views and priorities, until 1983 when America's first national health consumer organisation was formed. Well financed through a generous endowment by health book publisher, Rodale Press, the People's Medical

Society began life with a sophisticated strategy to enrol members in every state. Eventually the People's Medical Society reached 115,000 members, to become the largest consumer health organisation in America.

The goal of the organisation is to improve the quality of professional medical care through increasing public disclosure of relevant data; mobilising public political action at all levels of government; empowering individuals to take self protective action in the use of medical care; and investigating and reporting the competence of health care providers and institutions. I shall give only a few examples of the actions taken in these areas.

The People's Medical Society has promulgated or vigorously supported laws requiring hospitals to disclose publicly and routinely data on nosocomial infection rates, rates of diagnostic and treatment errors, frequency of surgical procedures, caesarean section and hysterectomy rates, and the status of malpractice law suits against hospital health care personnel. With regard to political action, the society mounts highly focused membership communications campaigns addressed at legislators. As many as 45,000 communications on behalf of (or opposed to) a piece of health legislation have been directed at legislators in a 48 hour period. These have been very effective in expanding access to information, in tightening up serious penalties for medical malfeasance, and in providing safeguards against alcohol and drug impaired physicians.

The society continued to press state governments to change from a physician licensure system to a certification system. This would include triannual written, oral and practical testing of all physicians and certifying only those skills where competence is demonstrated. No more lifetime licenses would be issued. A certification approach would help assist patients select practitioners according to specific competencies, regardless of the speciality label.[38] You can imagine the uproar this proposal is creating. On the other hand, during this tight budget period more and more legislatures are interested in saving the average of $400.00 cost of incompetent care which is now added to each hospital bill!

Central work of the society

The central work of the society, however, concentrates on individual empowerment. A physician evaluation form is completed by members after each office visit and filed by the society for reference by other members. The evaluation covers 20 aspects of the physician contact – for example waiting time, respect for patient integrity and privacy, quality of explanations provided, suggestions for self care and prevention, encouraging second opinions, etc. Physicians are invited to subscribe to the People's Medical Society 'Code of Good Practice' which entitles them to be entered in the society's recommended list of physicians.

Quality control, it seems is most effective at the point of medical contact. Members are encouraged when possible to take a relative or friend along to the doctor, or otherwise tape record the encounter for further review at a less stressful time. If the physician objects to the presence of a friend or relative, or tape recording, members are advised to see another physician, if this is feasible.

The society helps members prepare for medical encounters. Self protection guides are available with such titles as *Take this Book to the Hospital with you*,[39] *Take this Book to the Obstetrician with you*,[40] and *Take this Book to the Gynaecologist with you*.[41] Several members reported that merely placing a copy of the hospital book at the bedside had a positive effect on the care givers' attitudes and performance!

The People's Medical Society undertakes periodic assessments of hospitals through surveys of physicians and nurses practising in a given catchment area. The results of their preferences and the rankings of hospitals are published widely and serve to remind the public that quality, as judged by people who should know, varies among hospitals. It demonstrates the importance of being selective, of increasing choice.

Public participation in assuring quality of medical care in the USA has become serious business, tough and unrelenting in its process of discovery and demands for reform. It uncovers unpleasant facts about the real work of medical care and urgently challenges government and professionals to take action now. When it was seen, for example from the records of medical licensing boards in the 50 American states that only a tiny portion of malpracticing physicians are censured, much less barred from practice, the People's Medical Society began a campaign to make all membership on medical licensure and examining boards exclusively lay – no physicians – and to move to a jury system where expert medical and scientific witnesses could be heard. Lay representation also is being argued for on hospital medical and surgical audit teams. These are seen as necessary remedies in an environment where there is not now any built in system for public accountability.

The style of confrontation

You might have guessed that the style of the People's Medical Society is irreverent and provocative. This style, in itself, serves to communicate that it is alright, legal, ethical, and possible to criticise sacred cows openly and to challenge the conspiracy of silence within the health professions. Anger is a healthy emotion and fear of retribution is far less a threat to a person's well being that passivity in the face of doubtful medical competence. Those messages seem to be taking hold in an America where medical care was the last holdout against consumerism.

I am told by friends in Europe and Canada that a confrontational style is typically American. It would not work elsewhere, they say. Perhaps not. But one way or the other, the issues of information disclosure, equity, accountability, and empowerment will have to be addressed everywhere if we wish to achieve the promotion of health as envisioned in the Declaration of Alma Ata and in the World Health Organization's Ottawa Charter.[42] An initiative is now being considered in Hungary to organise a panEuropean association of health consumer organisations. Countries of central and eastern Europe and the newly independent states of the former Soviet Union present a propitious opportunity to develop a consumer voice in health. The optimistic view is that such an innovation can take root in this period of transition, where suspicion of government and authority in general runs high and the strategies of democracy are still novel and inviting.

The future

As chair of the board of directors of the People's Medical Society, and at the same time a long-time member of the public health establishment (and an academic at that!), I am well aware that an agenda of nihilism, doctor bashing, and general antiestablishmentism would be shallow, self-serving, and ultimately counterproductive. We must avoid replacing one tyranny with another. This can be accomplished by continuing to expand the partners in dialogue among public interest groups and the health professions where the partnership is mutually respectful. We should not misconstrue or be embarrassed by the passion in the voices on either side.

William Henry Duncan was nothing if he was not courageous. He took on the establishment with strong and persistent pressure. And he knew the value of a public constituency to move the political agenda.

Were he with us today, I believe he would be as undaunted in pursuit of solutions to problems from within the health professions and health system as he was in pursuit of problems within the community. He had to convince people of the environmental threat, its causes and its remedies, in the face of other beliefs and social priorities. I doubt he would tolerate any obstacle, not even his own professional identity, to bringing people around to a reasoned solution. We could use a little of that courage today in public health to evaluate our contribution to health on a full continuum from −1 to +1. Promoting health as Hippocrates emphasised, starts with doing no harm. Not a bad idea.

References

1. Arnstein S, as quoted in Schiller PL, Steckler A, Dawson L, Patton F. Participatory planning in community health education. Oakland, CA Third Party Publishing Company: 1987:20–21.
2. Carlson R, Newman B, eds. *Issues and trends in health.* St. Louis: CV Mosby, 1987.
3. Skrabanek P, McCormick J. *Follies and fallacies in medicine.* Buffalo, NY: Prometheus Books, 1990.
4. Round table discussions. *World Health Forum.* 1981;2(2): 191–201.
5. Friedson E. *Professional dominance: The social structure of medical care.* New York: Atherton Press, 1970.
6. Deria A. Self-Care puts the onus on the people themselves. *World Health Forum* 1981;12(2):194.
7. Katz AH, Levin LS. Self-care is not a solipsistic trap: A reply to critics. *Int J Health Serv* 1980;10:329–36.

8. Fry J. *Self-care, its place in the total health care system*. A report by an independent working party. London: Guy's Hospital, 1973:15.

9. Last J. The iceberg: Completing the clinical picture in general practice. *Lancet* 1963;ii:28–31.

10. Williamson JD, Danaher K. *Self-care in health*. London Croom-Helm, 1978.

11. Pratt L. The significance of the family in medication. *Journal of Comparative Family Studies*. 1973;4:13–31.

12. Freer CB. Self-care a health diary study. *Med Care* 1980; 18:853–61.

13. Elliott Binns, CP. An analysis of lay medicine. *JR Coll GP* 1973;23:255–64.

14. Alpert JJ, Kosa J, Haggerty RI. A month of illness and health care among low income families; *Public Health Rep* 1972;82:1004–12.

15. Zapka J, Averill BW. Self-care for colds: A cost effective alternative to upper respiratory infection management. *Am J Public Health* 1979;69:814–16.

16. Knapp DA, Knapp DE. Decision-making and self-medication: preliminary findings. *Am J Hospital Pharm* 1972; 29:1004–12.

17. Litman TJ. The family as a basic unit in health and medical care: A social-behavioural overview. *Soc Sci Med* 1974;53:495–519.

18. Katz HP, Clancy RR. Accuracy of home throat culture program: A study of parent participation in health care. *Paediatrics* 1974;53:687–91.

19. National Analysts Inc. *A study of health practices and opinions*. Springfield, VA: National Technical Information Service, US Department of Commerce; 1972, 343.

20. The Boston's Women's Health Book Collective. *Our bodies, ourselves*. New York: Simon and Schuster, 1971.

21. Carolyn De Marco. Medical malpractice. In: Hinks KM, ed. *Misdiagnosis: women as a disease*. Allentown: People's Medical Society, 1994:59.

22. Mendelsohn RS. *Confessions of a medical heretic*. Chicago: Warner Books, 1979.

23. Taylor R. *Medicine out of control*. Melbourne: Sun Books, 1979.

24. Rice S. *Some doctors make you sick*. Auckland: Angus and Robertson, 1988.

25. Skene Dust jacket: *You, your doctor and law*. Oxford University Press, Melbourne, 1990:IX.

26. Rachlis M, Kusher C. *Second Opinion*. Toronto; Collins, 1989.

27. Inlander C, Levin LS, Weiner E. *Medicine on trial*. New York: Prentice Hall Press, 1988:308.

28. Centre for Medical Consumers. *Health Facts*. 1990; XV(132):1,

29. Altman LK, Standard training in laparoscopy found inadequate. *New York Times*. Dec 14, 1993:C3.

30. Anonymous. Quality of care in the hospital. *People's Medical Society Newsletter* 1992; 11:1.

31. Vickery DM, Fries JF. *Take care of yourself*. Reading, MA: Addison-Wesley Publishing Company, 1986.

32. Simons A, Hasselbring B, Castleman M. *Before you call the doctor*. New York: Fawcett Columbine, 1992.

33. Howell M. *Healing at home*. Boston: Beacon Press, 1978.

34. Graedon J, Graedon T. *Graedon's best medicine: from herbal remedies to high tech Rx breakthroughs*. New York: Bantam Books, 1991.

35. Pelletier KR, *Holistic medicine: From stress to optimum health*. New York: Delacorte Press, 1979.

36. Belsky MS, Gross L. *How to choose and use your doctor*. New York: Arbor House, 1975, jacket.
37. Podell RN. *When your doctor doesn't know best*. New York: Simon and Schuster, 1994.
38. Andrews L. *Deregulating doctors*. Allentown, PA: People's Medical Society, 1986.
39. Inlander CB, Weiner E. *Take this book to the hospital with you*. New York: Pantheon Books, 1991.
40. Morales K, Inlander CB. *Take this book to the obstetrician with you*. Reading, MA: Addison-Wesley Publishing Inc, 1991.
41. Maleskey G, Inlander CB. *Take this book to the gynecologist with you*. Reading, MA: Addison-Wesley Publishing Inc, 1991.
42. *Ottawa charter for health promotion*. World Health Organization, Health and Welfare Canada, Canadian Public Health Association, No. 17–21, Ottawa, Canada, 1986.